Colonic Motility
From Bench Side to Bedside

Integrated Systems Physiology: from Molecule to Function to Disease

Editors

D. Neil Granger, *Louisiana State University Health Sciences Center-Shreveport*

Joey P. Granger, *University of Mississippi Medical Center*

Physiology is a scientific discipline devoted to understanding the functions of the body. It addresses function at multiple levels, including molecular, cellular, organ, and system. An appreciation of the processes that occur at each level is necessary to understand function in health and the dysfunction associated with disease. Homeostasis and integration are fundamental principles of physiology that account for the relative constancy of organ processes and bodily function even in the face of substantial environmental changes. This constancy results from integrative, cooperative interactions of chemical and electrical signaling processes within and between cells, organs, and systems. This eBook series on the broad field of physiology covers the major organ systems from an integrative perspective that addresses the molecular and cellular processes that contribute to homeostasis. Material on pathophysiology is also included throughout the eBooks. The state-of the-art treatises were produced by leading experts in the field of physiology. Each eBook includes stand-alone information and is intended to be of value to students, scientists, and clinicians in the biomedical sciences. Since physiological concepts are an ever-changing work-in-progress, each contributor will have the opportunity to make periodic updates of the covered material.

Published titles

(for future titles please see the Web site, www.morganclaypool.com/page/lifesci)

Colonic Motility: From Bench Side to Bedside
Sushil K. Sarna
www.morganclaypool.com

ISBN: 9781615041503 paperback

ISBN: 9781615041510 ebook

DOI: 10.4199/C00020ED1V01Y201011ISP011

A Publication in the Morgan & Claypool Publishers Life Sciences series

INTEGRATED SYSTEMS PHYSIOLOGY: FROM MOLECULE TO FUNCTION TO DISEASE

Book #11

Series Editors: D. Neil Granger, LSU Health Sciences Center, and Joey P. Granger, University of Mississippi Medical Center

Series ISSN Pending

Colonic Motility
From Bench Side to Bedside

Sushil K. Sarna
University of Texas Medical Branch

INTEGRATED SYSTEMS PHYSIOLOGY: FROM MOLECULE TO FUNCTION TO DISEASE #11

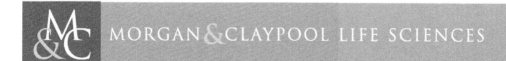

MORGAN&CLAYPOOL LIFE SCIENCES

ABSTRACT

Three distinct types of contractions perform colonic motility functions. Rhythmic phasic contractions (RPCs) cause slow net distal propulsion with extensive mixing/turning over. Infrequently occurring giant migrating contractions (GMCs) produce mass movements. Tonic contractions aid RPCs in their motor function. The spatiotemporal patterns of these contractions differ markedly. The amplitude and distance of propagation of a GMC are several-fold larger than those of an RPC. The enteric neurons and smooth muscle cells are the core regulators of all three types of contractions. The regulation of contractions by these mechanisms is modifiable by extrinsic factors: CNS, autonomic neurons, hormones, inflammatory mediators, and stress mediators. Only the GMCs produce descending inhibition, which accommodates the large bolus being propelled without increasing muscle tone. The strong compression of the colon wall generates afferent signals that are below nociceptive threshold in healthy subjects. However, these signals become nociceptive; if the amplitudes of GMCs increase, afferent nerves become hypersensitive, or descending inhibition is impaired. The GMCs also provide the force for rapid propulsion of feces and descending inhibition to relax the internal anal sphincter during defecation. The dysregulation of GMCs is a major factor in colonic motility disorders: irritable bowel syndrome (IBS), inflammatory bowel disease (IBD), and diverticular disease (DD). Frequent mass movements by GMCs cause diarrhea in diarrhea predominant IBS, IBD, and DD, while a decrease in the frequency of GMCs causes constipation. The GMCs generate the afferent signals for intermittent short-lived episodes of abdominal cramping in these disorders. Epigenetic dysregulation due to adverse events in early life is one of the major factors in generating the symptoms of IBS in adulthood.

KEYWORDS

smooth muscle, slow waves, enteric neurons, excitation-contraction coupling, peristaltic reflex, ICC, motility disorders, volume transmission, synaptic transmission, irritable bowel syndrome, inflammatory bowel disease, diverticular disease, diarrhea, constipation, visceral hypersensitivity, excitation-inhibition coupling, descending inhibition, abdominal pain, enteric nervous system, defecation, smooth muscle.

Dedication

I dedicate this work to my family, especially my parents, Dayal Saran Sarna and Nathi Devi Sarna, and my wife, Rajni Sarna, for their vision, dedication, guidance, sacrifices, and love.

Acknowledgments

I thank my teachers, students, colleagues and peers, who taught me what I know.

I am indebted to the National Institute of Diabetes and Digestive and Kidney Diseases, the Department of Veterans Affairs, the Canadian Institutes of Health, and the National Research Council Canada for generous research support over the years, which made this work possible.

In God I trust.

Contents

Introduction

MOTILITY REQUIREMENTS OF DIFFERENT ORGANS

Motility refers to spontaneous motion/movement, be it of a single cell moving through tissue or medium, or material moving inside hollow organs, e.g., the gastrointestinal tract, cardiovascular system, bladder, and uterus. In all cases, the cell or organ itself generates the force for motion. Cell motility results in its translocation or deformation of its membrane; organ motility results in mixing/turnover, propulsion, or both of the luminal contents. However, the rates of propulsion and the extent of mixing/turning-over vary among organs. Correspondingly, the modes of force generation differ among these organs. For the cardiovascular system, the primary movement is rapid and continuous blood circulation through a closed loop system. A single pump—the heart—performs this function by generating rhythmic phasic contractions (RPCs) sequentially in its four chambers. Myogenic mechanisms regulate the frequency and force of these contractions; circulating hormones and autonomic nerves may modulate them. Although numerous cell types and nutrients enter and leave the blood stream, blood consistency remains stable, and vigorous mixing movements are not required. The urinary bladder function requires storage until voluntary voiding. Tonic bladder smooth muscle contraction accompanied by centrally regulated sphincter relaxation accomplishes this function. The consistency of urine is also more or less constant.

The motility function of the gastrointestinal tract differs markedly from those of the cardiovascular system and the urinary bladder. First, the consistency and nature of ingested meals varies widely from liquid to solid. Second, numerous endocrine and exocrine secretions occur as the ingested meal moves through the gastrointestinal tract. These secretions digest the complex molecules in the meal into simpler molecules so they can be absorbed by the epithelial cells. The gut motility function requires thorough mixing of secretions with the ingested meal for complete digestion. In addition, the digesta needs frequent turnover to expose all of it uniformly to the epithelial surface for efficient absorption. Third, digestion and absorption are relatively slow processes, which require much slower but steady propulsion of digesta than that required by blood or urine. Therefore, the motility function of the gastrointestinal tract requires both mixing/turning over and propulsion of luminal contents. The propulsion of digesta generally occurs in irregular incremental steps, rather than in a continuous stream, as in cardiovascular circulation and bladder emptying. Further, digestive and absorptive functions are not constant throughout the gastrointestinal tract. The intensity of mixing/turning over and the rates of propulsion vary among the organs of the gastrointestinal tract, and in fact, in different parts of the same organ.

Little or no absorption of nutrients occurs in the esophagus, which is primarily a conduit for rapid transfer of the swallowed bolus from the upper esophageal sphincter to the gastric fundus without significant mixing/turning over. It takes less than 15 seconds for this transfer over about a 30-cm length of human esophagus.

The stomach secretes hydrochloric acid and pepsinogen for bacteriocidal action and protein digestion, respectively. Therefore, it requires mixing of these secretions with the meal, followed by slow and regulated emptying at a rate that does not overwhelm the digestive and absorptive capacity of the small intestine. Rapid gastric emptying results in malabsorption, while too-slow emptying may result in feelings of fullness, bloating, and nausea accompanied by weight loss. Accordingly, the motility function of the stomach is to store food temporarily in the gastric fundus, transfer it gradually to the corpus and the antrum, mix it with secretions, and triturate it in preparation for digestion in the small intestine. Coordinated motility of the antrum, pylorus, and duodenum empties the meal in small squirts into the small intestine. Hormonal, enteric neuronal, and extrinsic neuronal feedbacks stimulated by the nutrients entering the small intestine and sensory cells that monitor the state of digestion continuously modulate the gastric motility function for an optimal rate of gastric emptying. It takes about 15 to 30 minutes—called the lag phase of gastric emptying—for the stomach to begin emptying a solid meal into the small intestine. The lag phase is absent or short for liquid meals, which do not require trituration. The total gastric emptying time depends on the nutritional contents of the meal (carbohydrates, proteins, fat) and on meal viscosity.

Endocrine, pancreatic, and biliary secretions enter the proximal small intestine in response to meal ingestion. Most digestion and absorption of nutrients occurs in the proximal half of the small intestine. The bile acids are absorbed in the terminal ileum. Small intestinal motility intensively mixes the exocrine and endocrine secretions with the meal and at the same time spreads the mixture rapidly over the proximal half so that the entire absorptive surface is available for absorption of nutrients. The absorption rate of the bile acids is slower than that of the nutrients. As a result, the mixing function intensifies in the distal small intestine, while the propulsion rate slows. It takes about two hours for the head of an average meal to reach the ileocecal sphincter. The total small intestinal transit time depends on the nutritional content of the meal.

The digesta enters the colon as fluid. The colon absorbs most of the water and electrolytes for conservation and reduction of fecal mass. The colonic mucosa is tighter and its absorption rate slower than that of the small intestine. Therefore, it requires extensive turning over of its contents and a very slow net distal propulsion to absorb electrolytes and water. It takes over 24 hours for the digesta to move from the ileocecal sphincter to the rectum, a length of about one meter. In addition, the sigmoid colon and rectum serve as temporary storage for feces prior to defecation at a convenient and safe time. Although the colonic transit is ultraslow, ultrarapid propulsion accomplishes defecation in a short period.

Overall, propulsion rates slowdown as the ingested meal travels distally over the gastrointestinal tract, while the mixing/turning-over movements intensify. Such varied motility functions cannot be achieved by a single pump located at the beginning of the gastrointestinal tract, as in the cardiovascular system, or by individual pumps located at the beginning of each gut organ. Instead, smooth muscle cells at each location throughout the gut generate independent contractions. Through various enteric neural and myogenic regulatory mechanisms, these contractions organize as *propagating* and *nonpropagating* contractions of varying amplitudes and durations in response to sensory signals generated by local and distant conditions within the gut, to produce variable intensities of mixing/turning over and propulsion rates of the ingested meal.

Take-home Messages

1. Motility functions differ among different organs.
2. The motility function in the gut has two components: mixing/turning over and propulsion
3. The intensity of mixing and rates of propulsion differ between gut organs and often between different parts of the same organ.
4. The rate of propulsion of digesta decreases from the esophagus to the rectum, while the mixing/turning-over movements intensify.

HOW GUT CONTRACTIONS MIX/TURN OVER AND PROPEL DIGESTA

It is obvious that a single type of contraction, such as the more-or-less-constant-amplitude rhythmic phasic contractions of the cardiac muscle or the intermittent tonic contractions of the urinary bladder, could not perform the complex and varied motility functions of the gut. The propulsion of digesta in the gut does not occur by creating a pressure differential between adjacent organs or between the oral and anal ends of a short segment. Instead, the digesta is propelled when the contractions propagate, similar to propulsion by a peristaltic pump, where each stroke of the piston propels. The efficacies of mixing/turning over and propulsion depend on the spatiotemporal characteristics of contractions.

The temporal characteristics of gut contractions include frequency, amplitude, and duration, whereas the spatial characteristics include direction of propagation, distance of propagation, and velocity of propagation. These spatiotemporal characteristics of contractions determine whether they (1) propel, (2) produce back and forth movements to mix, stir, and turn over the fecal material, or (3) do both [1–5].

Each smooth muscle cell in the gut wall generates independent contractions. However, communication between adjacent smooth muscle cells through gap junctions and neuronal networks in the myenteric and submucosal plexi coordinates contractions spatially to varying degrees in different parts of the gut. This coordination allows some contractions to occur sequentially at adjacent locations to various distances in the gut (*propagating contractions*), while others do not propagate or propagate over very short distances (*nonpropagating contractions*). Input from the cholinergic excitatory motor neurons and the excitation-contraction coupling in smooth muscle cells (see later) determine the amplitudes of propagating and nonpropagating contractions. The amplitude of a contraction and its distance of propagation together determine the distance a single bolus of digesta is propelled by each propagating contraction.

Figure 1A illustrates a contraction beginning at a proximal location and propagating in the anal direction. This contraction is strong to occlude the lumen. As a result, it propels the digesta trapped ahead of it up to the distance of its propagation, at the same time causing modest mixing. The speed of propulsion of the bolus of digesta is nearly the same as the velocity of propagation of the contraction. The frequency of propagated contractions determines the total volume of digesta propelled per unit of time. The lumen-occluding propagating contractions occur frequently in the gastric antrum and in the proximal small intestine. The contraction in Figure 1B also propagates, but it is not strong enough to occlude the lumen. A part of the digesta escapes through the luminal opening as the contraction propagates and is left behind to cause mixing. This type of contraction is less propulsive than that in Figure 1A; however, it produces more mixing. This type of contraction occurs in the gastric corpus and mid small intestine. The contractions in Figure 1C occur randomly at adjacent locations; some occlude the lumen, while others do not. These nonpropagating contractions produce back and forth movements of the digesta, causing intense mixing/turning over with slow net distal propulsion. These types of contractions occur predominantly in the terminal ileum and the colon. The contraction shown in Figure 1D is also a lumen-occluding propagating contraction like that in Figure 1A. However, this contraction is much stronger in amplitude and longer in duration, and it propagates uninterrupted over several-fold longer distances than the one in Figure 1A. Such contractions are ultrapropulsive. They cause mass movements, such as those during defecation.

Take-home Messages

1. The spatiotemporal characteristics of gut contractions determine their efficacy in mixing/turning over and propulsion of digesta.
2. The spatiotemporal characteristics are different in each organ of the gut.

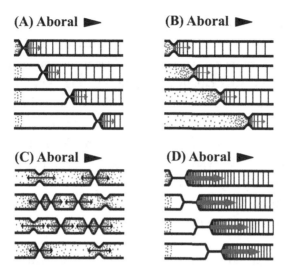

FIGURE 1: The role of different spatiotemporal patterns of contractions in mixing and propulsion in the gut. (A) A lumen-occluding contraction that propagates in the anal direction propels the digesta ahead of it up to the distance of its propagation. The gastric antrum and proximal small intestine generally generate this type of contractions. (B) A contraction that only partially occludes the lumen and propagates causes some propulsion and some mixing. The gastric corpus and most of the small intestine generate this type of contraction. (C) Spatially disorganized contractions that may or may not occlude the lumen cause much mixing with very little propulsion. The terminal ileum and the entire colon generate this type of contraction. (D) A large-amplitude, long-duration, and rapidly propagating contraction, occludes a long segment of the gut and is highly effective in propulsion of digesta. The esophagus generates this type of contraction with each swallow. The terminal ileum and the proximal colon generate this type of contraction infrequently. This type of contraction precedes normal defecation.

TYPES OF GUT CONTRACTIONS

Gut smooth muscle cells generate three distinct types of contractions which together achieve the complex and varied mixing and propulsive functions of the gut: (1) rhythmic phasic contractions (RPCs), (2) ultrapropulsive contractions (UPCs), and (3) tonic contractions (TCs). A gut smooth muscle cell can generate concurrently all three types of contractions.

Rhythmic Phasic Contractions

RPCs (Figure 1A, B, and C) are the workhorse of the postprandial gut motility function. They cause slow net distal propulsion and mixing/turnover of the ingested meal. These contractions occur in the stomach, small intestine, and the colon after a meal as well as during the interdigestive state.

Ultrapropulsive Contractions

UPCs (Figure 1D) are of two types: giant migrating contractions (GMCs) and retrograde giant contractions (RGCs). These contractions are several-fold larger in amplitude and longer in duration than RPCs (Figure 2). The GMCs rapidly propagate (~1 cm/sec) in the anal direction over very long distances [6]. The RGCs originate in the mid small intestine and rapidly propagate (~10 cm/sec) in the oral direction up to the antrum [7] (Figure 3). Both types of giant contractions produce mass movements, i.e., rapid propulsion of luminal contents over long segments of the gut. The rapid transit caused by GMCs and RGCs does not allow much contact time between the digesta and the mucosal surface, precluding any digestion or absorption during the mass movement.

GMCs are more effective than RPCs in propulsion because of the marked differences in the spatiotemporal characteristics of these two types of contractions.

1. Propagating RPCs are not always strong enough to occlude the lumen. However, the amplitude of GMCs is twofold to threefold larger than that of the largest RPCs [6], and therefore, GMCs invariably occlude the lumen.
2. GMCs last several-fold longer than RPCs, helping them easily overcome any resistance in the propulsion of luminal contents.

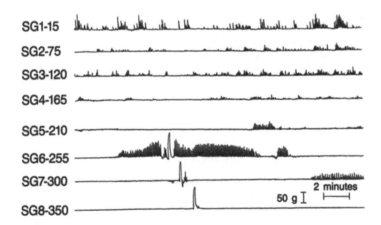

FIGURE 2: Record showing a small intestinal GMC starting in the middle of a migrating motor complex, propagating in the anal direction at the strain gauge transducer SG6—implanted surgically at 255 cm from the pylorus. Note the much larger amplitude and longer duration of the GMC compared with spontaneous RPCs occurring at different strain gauge transducers. The GMC propagated to the last transducer SG8 located 95 cm away in about 2 minutes. SG = strain gauge transducer. Numbers after dashes indicate the distance of the transducer in cm from the pylorus.

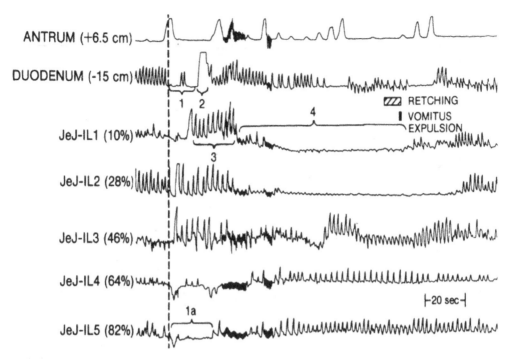

FIGURE 3: Record showing an RGC starting at strain gauge transducer Jej-IL3 located at 46% of the length of the small bowel from the pylorus. Note the larger amplitude and longer duration of RGC and its rapid propagation to the antrum (~10 cm/sec). Retching and vomiting followed the oral propagation of RGC, which regurgitated the luminal contents of the proximal half of the small intestine into the stomach in preparation for vomiting. Jej = jejunum, IL = Ileum. Percentages after these symbols indicate the location of the transducers as a percentage of the total length of the small intestine. (Reproduced with permission from Lang, IM, Sarna, SK, and Condon, RE, *Gastroenterology*, 90(1): 40–47, 1986 [7].)

3. A propagating RPC usually propagates a few centimeters at a time. By contrast, a GMC propagates over appreciable distances and often to the end of the organ in which it origi- nates [6].

In humans and most nonrodent species, GMCs occur spontaneously in the small intestine and the colon [6, 8–10]. In the distal small intestine, they occur primarily in the fasting state after digestion is complete. However, in the colon, they occur in the fasting and the postprandial state. In the esophagus, a swallow stimulates a GMC that propagates in the anal direction. It strongly compresses the esophageal wall, relaxing the lower esophageal sphincter by descending inhibition to let the bolus pass through (Figure 4) [11]. Reflux of gastric contents also can stimulate GMCs in the distal esophagus to clear the esophagus rapidly (secondary peristalsis).

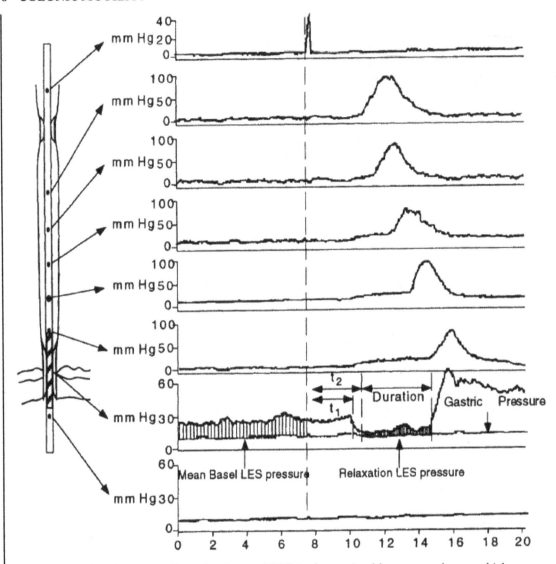

FIGURE 4: A voluntary swallow stimulates a GMC in the proximal human esophagus, which propagates in the anal direction and induces descending inhibition of the lower esophageal tone to let the swallowed bolus pass through without resistance. A manometric catheter, shown on the left side, recorded the contractions. (Reproduced with permission from Shi et al. and Kahrilas, PJ, *Am J Gastroenterol*, 93: 2373–2379, 1998 [11].)

Species such as rodents, guinea pigs, and rabbits defecate compacted pellets instead of the formed stools produced by higher species such as humans and dogs. These pellets form in the midcolon, proximal to which the fecal material is thick fluid. Since colonic RPCs are not powerful enough to propel hard pellets effectively, the colons in these species generate predominantly GMCs [12–18]. GMCs in the rat colon occur at a frequency of about 17 to 45/hour [12] and in the mouse colon at about 15 to 25/hour [15] (Figure 5). However, unlike in human and canine colons, most GMCs in the rodent colon do not always propagate or propagate only over short distances and hence are responsible for the gradual distal propulsion of the pellets [12].

Tonic Contractions

The circular smooth muscle cells of the sphincters (the lower esophageal sphincter and the internal anal sphincter) and organ junctions (the pylorus and ileocecal junction) in the gut generate a sustained tonic contraction, which keeps their lumen partially or completely closed to prevent reflux.

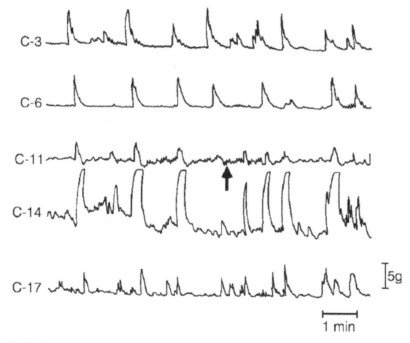

FIGURE 5: Colonic motor activity in an intact conscious rat. The colon generated primarily GMCs. Arrow shows tiny RPCs. C = colonic strain gauge transducer. The number after C indicates the distance in cm of the transducer from the cecum. (Reproduced with permission from Li et al. and Sarna, SK, *Am J Physiol Gastrointest Liver Physiol*, 283: G544–G552, 2002 [12].)

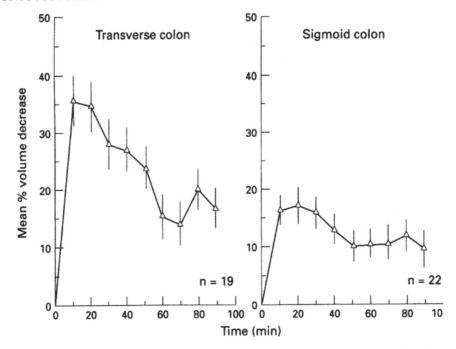

FIGURE 6: Increase of circular muscle tone in the human transverse and sigmoid colon after ingestion of a meal. A barostat recorded the tone. The increase of tone reduces the volume inside the balloon to maintain it at a constant pressure. The increase of postprandial tone is greater in the transverse colon than in the sigmoid colon. (Reproduced with permission from Ford et al. and Camilleri, M, *Gut*, 37(2): 264–269, 1995 [20].)

Activation of enteric inhibitory neurons reduces this tone to allow the passage of luminal contents in the distal direction.

The smooth muscle cells in the major organs also generate a basal tone that maintains their resting shape in length and diameter. The ingestion of a meal increases the tone of circular muscle cells in the small intestine and the colon, which narrows the lumen to varying degrees but does not occlude it [19–21] (Figure 6). The amplitude and duration of increase in tone depend upon the volume and caloric intake of food [20]. The generation of tone by itself does not cause major mixing/turnover or propulsion; however, it narrows the lumen to accentuate the motility function of RPCs. With a narrower lumen, weaker RPCs, such as those shown in Figure 1B, might occlude the lumen to enhance their effectiveness in propulsion and/or mixing/turning over.

Take-home Messages

1. The gut generates three distinct types of contractions, rhythmic phasic contractions (RPCs);

ultrapropulsive contractions (UPCs), which are of two types, giant migrating contractions (GMCs) and retrograde giant contractions (RGCs); and tonic contractions (TCs).

2. Each type of contraction plays a distinct role in the mixing/turning over and propulsive roles of gut motility function.

DESCENDING INHIBITION

Due to their strong lumen-occluding amplitude and long distances of uninterrupted propagation, GMCs propel a large bolus of digesta in the segment over which they propagate. The bolus accumulates in size as the GMC propagates, causing distension of the receiving segment. In healthy subjects, the distal segment relaxes its tone and inhibits its ongoing RPCs (Figure 7), thus accommodating the large bolus without generating resistance against propulsion. This is called descending inhibition [8–10, 22]. It is stimulated by strong compression of the gut wall by a GMC,

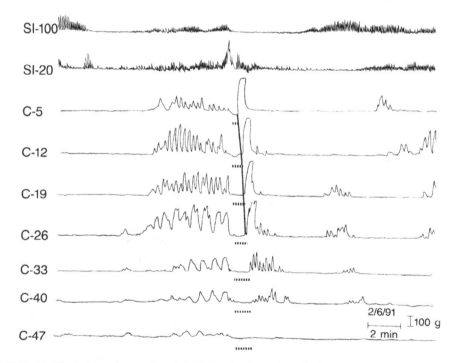

FIGURE 7: GMCs induce descending inhibition in the colon. A GMC originated at the location of strain gauge transducer C5 (5 cm distal to the ileocecal junction) and propagated in the anal direction up to the location of transducer C26 (26 cm distal to the ileocecal junction). Dotted lines show descending inhibition of spontaneous ongoing contractions. C = colonic strain gauge transducer, SI = small intestinal strain gauge transducer. The numbers after these symbols indicate the distance in cm of the transducers from the ileocecal junction. (Reproduced with permission from Otterson et al. and Sarna, SK, *Am J Physiol [Gastrointest Liver Physiol]*, 26: G518–G526, 1992 [420].)

stimulating in turn descending interneurons which themselves connect to inhibitory motor neurons projecting into smooth muscle cells [9, 23]. The descending inhibition also relaxes the tone of the sphincters—the lower esophageal sphincter and internal anal sphincter—for easy passage of the large bolus through them [10, 11].

Bayliss and Starling [24] initially used the term peristalsis to describe a contraction that begins above a local luminal stimulus and propagates distally while producing descending inhibition of spontaneous contractions and relaxation of tone ahead of it. As noted above, GMCs meet these conditions [6, 8–10] but not RPCs [1, 3, 25]. Note that RPCs do not induce descending inhibition (Figure 7), because they do not strongly compress the gut wall, and they do not propagate over long distances to accumulate a large bolus. Instead, they propel digesta in small amounts over short distances, which may fill the receiving segment and shift luminal contents back and forth but does not distend it. The original term "peristalsis", therefore, applies only to GMCs.

Take-home Messages

1. Among the three types of gut contractions, only GMCs produce descending inhibition. The strong compression of the gut wall initiates the descending inhibitory signal.
2. RPCs are not strong enough to initiate the descending inhibitory signal.

COMPOSITION OF THREE TYPES OF CONTRACTIONS IN GUT ORGANS

The composition of the three types of contractions differs among the gut organs to meet their specific requirements of motility function, that is, the rate of propulsion and intensity of mixing/turning over. The esophageal muscles generate predominantly GMCs that rapidly propel the swallowed bolus from the pharyngeal sphincter into the stomach without any mixing, because no digestion/absorption occurs in this organ. The gastric fundus serves as a temporary reservoir to hold the ingested meal. It relaxes (adaptive relaxation) to accommodate the large volume of ingested meal. Thereafter, it generates a slowly rising tonic contraction that gradually transfers the meal to the corpus, where the mixing and propulsive movements begin [5]. The gastric corpus and antrum generate primarily RPCs to mix the ingested meal with acid and pepsinogen secretions. The amplitude of a gastric RPC increases as it propagates from the corpus to the antrum. Under appropriate antropyloroduodenal coordination, a small bolus of the ingested meal empties into the duodenum with each propagating gastric RPC.

The small intestine generates all three types of contractions. Its tone increases after a meal to narrow the lumen [21]. Intestinal RPCs cause mixing/turnover and slow net distal propulsion of the digesta. The percentage of small intestinal postprandial RPCs that propagate and the mean distance of their propagation decrease from the duodenum to the terminal ileum, which accounts for the decrease in propulsion rate and the intensification of mixing/turning over from the duodenum to the ileum [1, 2, 25, 26]. In healthy individuals, the few GMCs in the small intestine occur in the terminal ileum to empty rapidly any material refluxed from the proximal colon to the terminal ileum [27].

In practice, GMCs can start anywhere in the small intestine and propagate uninterruptedly to the terminal ileum. In extreme cases of rapid propulsion, a GMC may begin in the distal small intestine and propagate uninterruptedly all the way to the anal sphincter to expel the entire contents of the distal small intestine and the colon within a few minutes. The small intestine also generates RGCs, which rapidly retropel the contents of the proximal half of the small intestine into the stomach in preparation for vomiting [7]. RGCs occur in response to ingestion of a noxious substance or in response to a central stimulus. RGCs invariably start in the mid small intestine and propagate uninterruptedly to the antrum. RGCs may not start distal to the mid small intestine, probably due to regurgitation of unpleasant digesta in the distal small intestine and because it may be just as easy to rapidly expel the digesta from these locations via the colon by GMCs. In contrast to the stomach and the small intestine, the colon generates only RPCs, GMCs, and TCs. The following section discusses the roles of these types of contractions in colonic motility function.

Take-home Messages

1. The composition of the three types of contractions differs among the major organs in the gut. The esophagus generates primarily GMCs.
2. The stomach generates RPCs and tonic contractions only.
3. The small intestine generates RPCs, TCs, RGCs, and GMCs.
4. The colon generates RPCs, TCs, and GMCs only.
5. Numerous terminologies and classifications of contractions exist in the literature on gut motor activity, specifically for GMCs. One publication lists seven different types of contractions in the colon [28]; others define contractions based on their amplitude, duration, or propagation. The author recognizes that no terminology is perfect. This book uses a terminology that defines minimum types of contractions based on their regulatory mechanisms. A simple terminology that relates description of contractions to their regulatory mechanisms might help bridge the gap between basic science and clinical studies. "Giant" in "giant migrating contractions" and "retrograde giant contractions" refers to disproportionately larger amplitude, duration, and distance of propagation of these contractions.

FUNCTIONS AND SPATIOTEMPORAL CHARACTERISTICS OF COLONIC CONTRACTIONS

The colon is the final major organ in the gastrointestinal tract. Its motility function has a major impact on the frequency and timing of defecation as well as on the consistency and shape of stools.

These variables differ markedly between species. For example, both humans and dogs normally defecate once or twice a day and have formed feces. On the other hand, rodents and guinea pigs—used frequently in experimental studies—defecate frequently and produce pellets. Consequently, the composition of the above three types of colonic contractions differs between species. In addition, the spatiotemporal characteristics of the same type of contraction differ in the colons of different species. For example, GMCs occur only a few times a day in human and dog colons, but in rodent colons, these contractions occur frequently but irregularly [12–18]. It is, therefore, crucial to identify the type of contraction to evaluate colonic motor function and investigate its mechanisms of regulation by species. Failure to do so would make it difficult to extrapolate the findings from animal models to human colonic motility function in health and disease and may lead to contradictory results because the regulatory mechanisms of different types of colonic contractions differ. For example, slow waves regulate the maximum frequency and timing of RPCs, but they do not regulate these characteristics in GMCs and TCs.

The colon wall, like the rest of the gut, has two outer muscle layers: the circular muscle layer and the longitudinal muscle layer. In humans, the longitudinal muscle layer is bundled into three-taenia coli with a thin longitudinal muscle coat over the rest of the surface. In other species, such as dogs, the longitudinal muscle layer is a thin uniform coat around the circumference. The contractions of the circular muscle cells partially or completely occlude the lumen, and hence, they are effective in mixing, turning over, and propulsion as they propagate. Contractions of the longitudinal muscle shorten the length of the colon, which has minimal effect on mixing and propulsive functions. For this reason, the following sections do not discuss longitudinal muscle contractions.

Colonic Rhythmic Phasic Contractions

The spatiotemporal characteristics of RPCs, which cause the postprandial function of mixing/turn-over and net distal propulsion, differ between organs. For example, the maximum frequency of contractions in the human stomach is about 3 times per minute, in the duodenum about 12 times per minute, which decreases to about 6 to 8 times per minute in the ileum. The digesta in the stomach and the small intestine is largely fluid. By contrast, the fluid contents of the ascending colon gradually become semisolid to solid in the sigmoid colon as water is absorbed. To meet the challenge of turning over and slowly propelling the semisolid to solid contents, the colon generates two types of RPCs, short-duration RPCs (2 to 3 seconds in duration) and long-duration RPCs (15 to 20 seconds) [29–31] (Figure 8). The short-duration contractions show little or no propagation, and their amplitudes vary considerably. The long-duration contractions may propagate over short distances [29]. The longer duration of long-duration RPCs enables them to turn over and propel the semisolid to solid contents more effectively. The frequency of short-duration RPCs in the human colon is about 3 to 12 times per minute; that of long-duration RPCs is about 0.5 to 2 times per minute.

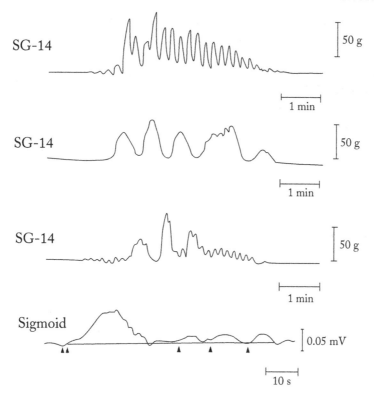

FIGURE 8: Short- and long-duration contractions in canine and human colons. The top tracing shows short-duration RPCs in the dog colon. The second tracing shows long-duration RPCs. The third tracing from the top shows three long-duration RPCs followed by a series of short-duration RPCs. The same strain gauge transducer (SG14) located at 14 cm distal to the ileocolonic junction made all three recordings. The bottom tracing shows a long-duration RPC followed by a series of short-duration RPCs recorded by a manometric tube from the human sigmoid colon.

Short-duration RPCs occur more frequently, while long-duration RPCs occur in bursts generally lasting a few minutes [29, 30]. The variability in the frequency of colonic RPCs is much greater than that of gastric and small intestinal RPCs. Together, colonic RPCs are highly disorganized in space and vary widely in amplitude and duration, making them effective in turning over of fecal material with a very slow rate of propulsion. Different mechanisms regulate these two types of phasic contractions, as discussed later.

The rodent colon also generates RPCs, but their amplitude in the intact conscious state is very small when recorded by strain gauge transducers [12, 15, 18]. The feces, already semisolid in the proximal rat colon, form discrete hard pellets in the middle and distal colons. The small-amplitude

RPCs are unlikely to affect significantly the mixing or propulsion of these contents. Instead, the rodent colon generates frequent GMCs [12, 13, 32], as discussed in the next section.

Colonic Giant Migrating Contractions

Giant migrating contractions (GMCs) in the human and canine colons are large-amplitude lumen-occluding contractions that propagate very rapidly (about 1 cm/sec) in the distal direction over appreciable distances to produce mass movements [8, 22, 28, 33–40]. In these species, spontaneous GMCs occur randomly about 2 to 10 times a day in the proximal, middle, or descending segments of the colon. Colonic GMCs occur in both the fasting and the postprandial state.

Take-home Messages

1. RPCs in the colon are of two types, short-duration and long-duration. Short-duration RPCs mostly turn over the fecal material. Long-duration RPCs propagate over short distances and produce mild propulsion.
2. GMCs occur up to about 10 times per 24 hours in healthy humans. They produce mass movements and provide the force for expulsion of feces during defecation.

·   ·   ·   ·

Regulatory Mechanisms

The generation of gut contractions and their organization into spatiotemporal patterns that result in propagating and nonpropagating contractions is autonomous. Specifically, input from the extrinsic nerves or hormones is not required to generate or organize them. The smooth muscle cells and the enteric neurons are the core cell types that together regulate motility function autonomously (Figure 9). However, input from external sources (sympathetic and parasympathetic neurons; paracrine,

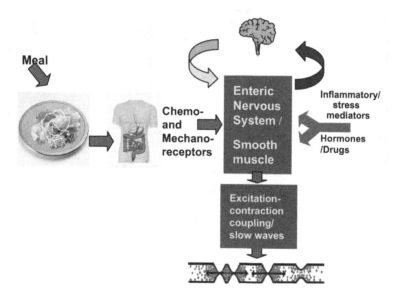

FIGURE 9: An overview of the regulation of gut motility functions in health and in disease. The presence of a meal in the lumen activates chemoreceptors and mechanoreceptors, which send appropriate signals to the enteric nervous system. The enteric nervous system maintains bidirectional communication with the brain via the autonomic nerves (gut-brain axis). The brain monitors the gut function to modulate its behavior, as necessary. The enteric motor neurons release excitatory and inhibitory neurotransmitters in response to afferent signals from the mucosal sensory receptors. The smooth muscle cells generate slow waves and initiate excitation-contraction and excitation-inhibition couplings in response to excitatory and inhibitory neurotransmitters. The enteric neurons and smooth muscle cells together regulate the type of contraction generated and its spatiotemporal organization.

endocrine, and exocrine hormones; inflammatory mediators or stress mediators) may influence the myogenic and enteric neuronal regulation to modify the characteristics of gut contractions in response to changes in the external environment. The autonomic nerves do not directly innervate the smooth muscle cells. Instead, they modulate the activity of the enteric nervous system, which, in turn, affects the overall motility function.

Figure 10 shows the roles of the enteric nervous system and circular smooth muscle cells in regulating gut contractions in the presence of digesta/feces in the lumen. The sensory nerve endings

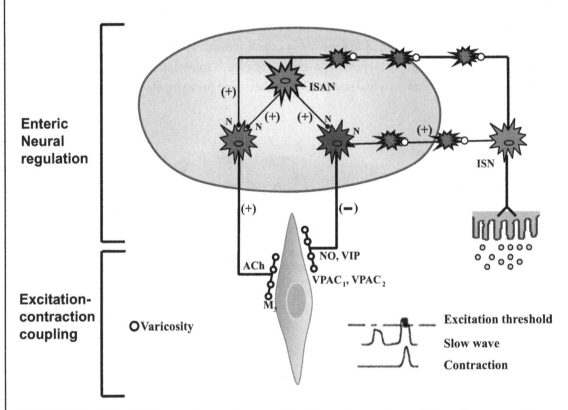

FIGURE 10: A detailed view of the enteric neuronal and smooth muscle regulation of gut contractions. The digesta activates enterochromaffin (EC) cells to releases 5-HT, which activates 5-HT$_4$ receptors on mucosal sensory nerve endings. The sensory nerve endings transmit the signal to the motor neurons via the interneurons. CGRP and ACh serve as neurotransmitters of the sensory neurons. The interneurons synapse on excitatory and inhibitory motor neurons to release ACh and NO, respectively. These neurotransmitters activate the excitation-contraction and excitation-inhibition couplings shown in Figure 11. Intrinsic spontaneously active neurons (ISANs) show spontaneous activity in the absence of any digesta in the lumen. These neurons synapse on motor neurons to release excitatory and inhibitory motor neurotransmitters, stimulating contractions in the absence of digesta.

in the mucosal surface detect the chemical composition and presence of nutrients by chemoreceptors and mechanoreceptors, respectively. The interneurons convey this information to the excitatory and inhibitory motor neurons in the myenteric ganglia. Note that this figure shows only a single ganglion. The myenteric ganglia organize as a two-dimensional network of interconnected ganglia covering the circumference and length of the gastrointestinal tract [41]. Therefore, in practice, the luminal contents at a given location will send the signal to several ganglia within the sphere of influence of the sensory receptors stimulated by them. The area of influence may include ganglia both proximal and distal to the segment directly in contact with the digesta.

On stimulation, the excitatory and inhibitory motor neurons release neurotransmitters, which respectively induce excitation-contraction and excitation-inhibition couplings in smooth muscle cells (Figure 10). Acetylcholine (ACh) is the established physiological excitatory neurotransmitter of gut contractions in the intact state; atropine, a nonspecific antagonist of muscarinic receptors, blocks in vivo gut contractions [42–45]. Substance P (SP) colocalizes with ChAT-immunoreactive neurons and stimulates in vitro colonic contractions [46]. However, we do not know whether tachykinin receptor antagonists block spontaneous colonic contractions in intact animals. In vitro studies show that SP mediates gut contractions in response to larger intraluminal stimuli [47, 48].

Nitric oxide (NO) is the physiological neurotransmitter of intrinsic inhibitory motor neurons and descending inhibition [49–51]. Vasoactive intestinal polypeptide (VIP) colocalizes with nNOS in inhibitory motor neurons. However, VIP antagonism does not block descending inhibition in intact animals [23]. SP and VIP are potential candidates as excitatory and inhibitory neurotransmitters; however, their precise roles in colonic motor function remain unknown. Recent studies found a novel role of VIP: it induces excitation-transcription coupling in gut smooth muscle cells to enhance expression of the pore-forming α_{1C} subunit of L-type calcium channels (see section on excitation-transcription coupling). The following sections discuss the complementary roles of smooth muscle cells and enteric neurons in generating the three types of colonic contractions.

RHYTHMIC PHASIC CONTRACTIONS
Short-Duration Rhythmic Phasic Contractions
Excitation-Contraction Coupling. The smooth muscle cells contain actin (thin filament) and myosin (thick filament). Myosin is a hexamer comprised of two paired 230-kDa heavy chains. Each chain is composed of a head (cross-bridge); a tail; and two light chains, a 20-kDa regulatory light chain (RLC_{20}) and a 17-kDa essential light chain. These muscle cells contract when actin and myosin filaments interact by cross-bridge cycling [52, 53]. In the resting state, the binding of ATP to the myosin head dissociates it from actin (released state). Phosphorylation of RLC_{20} hydrolyses ATP to ADP by ATPase activity and releases phosphate. The released energy cocks the myosin head to a new position on the actin chain (cross-bridge state). The release of phosphate changes the myosin

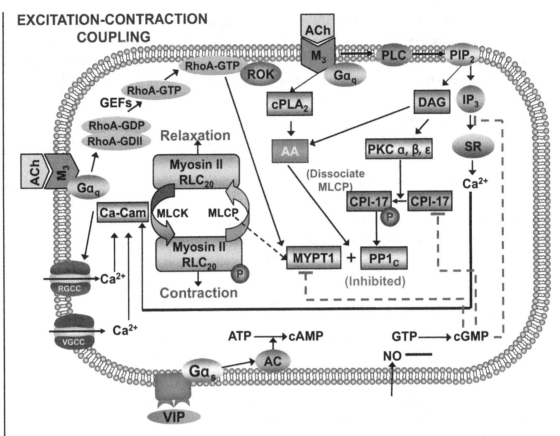

FIGURE 11: Signaling pathways for generating the three types of contractions in colonic circular smooth muscle cells. The electromechanical coupling initiated by slow-wave depolarization induces an influx of Ca^{2+} through voltage-gated calcium channels (L-type or $Ca_v1.2b$ channels). The binding of ACh to muscarinic M_3 receptors initiates multiple signaling pathways that induce further Ca^{2+} influx through receptor-gated Ca^{2+} channels; release intracellular Ca^{2+} from IP$_3$-sensitive stores; inhibit MLCP; and increase the phosphorylation of MLC$_{20}$ via PKC, ROK, and release of AA to enhance the amplitude and/or duration of contraction, resulting in the generation of three types of contractions. GEFs = guanine nucleotide exchange factors; CaM = calmodulin; MYPT1 and PP1c = regulatory and catalytic subunits, respectively, of MLCP (myosin light chain phosphatase); CPI-17 = PKC-potentiated inhibitor protein of 17 kDa; AA = arachidonic acid; PKC = protein kinase C; DAG = diacylglycerol; SR = sarcoplasmic reticulum; PIP$_2$ = phosphatidyl inositon 4,5,-biphosphate; PLC = phospholipase C; IP$_3$ = inositol 1,4,5-triphosphate; cPLA$_2$ = cytosolic phospholipase A$_2$; MLCK = myosin light chain kinase; RhoGDI = GDP dissociation inhibitor; ROK = Rho kinase; ACh = acetylcholine.

head conformation to cock it into a new position on the actin chain (cross-bridge state), resulting in force generation and sliding of myosin and actin filaments past each other to cause cell shortening. The amplitude and duration of cell shortening depend on the degree and duration of cross-bridge cycling, which in turn depends on the intensity and duration of RLC_{20} phosphorylation. Myosin light chain kinase (MLCK) phosphorylates RLC_{20}, resulting in cell contraction, whereas myosin light chain phosphatase (MLCP) dephosphorylates it, resulting in its return to the basal state (Figure 11).

The binding of cytosolic free calcium to calmodulin activates MLCK (Figure 11). Mammalian MLCP is a trimeric enzyme consisting of a catalytic 37- to 38-kDa subunit PP1c, an associated 110- to 130-kDa regulatory targeting subunit MYPT1, and a tightly bound 20-kDa subunit of unknown function [54–56]. MYPT1, through its NH_2 terminus, binds the MLCP complex to myosin II and enhances the catalytic activity of PP1c. The dephosphorylation rate of myosin II decreases when (1) the subunits of MLCP-MYPT1 and PP1c dissociate, (2) the catalytic activity of PP1c decreases, or (3) the binding activity of MYPT1 decreases by phosphorylation (or thiophosphorylation) of Thr-696.

RLC_{20} is phosphorylated constitutively in the resting state of smooth muscle cells due to a low concentration of cytosolic free Ca^{2+} (70 to 100 nM) that maintains the basal tone. In this state, the rates of basal phosphorylation of RLC_{20} by MLCK and dephosphorylation by MLCP are maintained in equilibrium. The cell contracts if MLCK activity increases, MLCP activity decreases, or both occur concurrently. The cell returns to its resting state when MLCK activity decreases or MLCP activity increases. The excitation-contraction coupling in gut smooth muscle cells has two components: *electromechanical coupling* and *pharmacomechanical coupling*.

Electromechanical Coupling. Electromechanical coupling results from the spontaneous periodic depolarization of colonic circular smooth muscle cells, called slow wave. Each slow-wave depolarization consists of three major components: upstroke, plateau, and repolarization potentials (Figure 12A). The generation of slow waves is insensitive to L-type calcium channel blockers. However, we do not know the precise ionic mechanisms of their spontaneous initiation. The colonic smooth muscle cells have a resting membrane potential of about −60 to −80 mV [57–60]. The membrane depolarization during plateau potential is in the range of −40 mV to −50 mV. This depolarization induces Ca^{2+} influx by opening the voltage-gated calcium channels (L-type or $Ca_v1.2b$) [61]. As indicated above, the resulting increase in cytosolic free Ca^{2+} binds with calmodulin to activate MLCK and phosphorylate RLC_{20}. However, current-voltage curves obtained by patch clamping of colonic smooth muscle cells show that these channels conduct very little calcium current in the membrane potential range of −40 mV to −50 mV [62] (Figure 12B). Therefore, the slow-wave depolarization by itself is below the threshold for generating RPCs that can mix/turn over and propel luminal

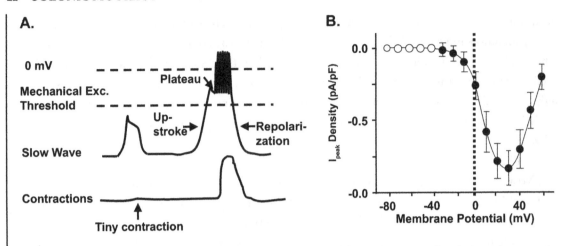

A.

0 mV

Plateau

Mechanical Exc.
Threshold

Up-
stroke →   ← Repolari-
zation

Slow Wave

Contractions

↑
Tiny contraction

B.

I_{peak} Density (pA/pF)

0.0

-0.5

-0.0

-80   -40   0   40
Membrane Potential (mV)

FIGURE 12: Slow wave and smooth muscle contraction. (A) The slow wave depolarizes the smooth muscle membrane in the range of about −40mV to −50 mV from a resting membrane potential in the range of −60 mV to −80 mV. However, as shown in (B), this depolarization induces very small inward calcium current (electromechanical coupling). Therefore, slow-wave depolarization by itself generates a very tiny contraction. Any ACh released during the slow-wave depolarization induces additional calcium influx through calcium channels as well as calcium release from the endoplasmic stores. In addition, the cell-signaling pathways initiated by the binding of ACh to muscarinic M_3 receptors increases calcium sensitivity to further enhance contraction amplitude (pharmacomechanical coupling). The electromechanical and pharmacomechanical couplings together (see Figure 11) generate the postprandial contractions, which are of sufficient amplitude and duration to cause mixing/turning over and propulsion of the digesta. (Reproduced with permission from Sarna, SK, *Am J Physiol Gastrointest Liver Physiol*, 294: 372–390, 2008 [79].)

contents [62, 63] (Figure 12). It results in a tiny contraction that is largely ineffective in mixing or propulsion. In vivo recordings barely record the contractions resulting only due to Ca^{2+} influx by slow-wave depolarization.

In vitro recordings of isolated circular smooth muscle strips or full-thickness rings of the colon in organ bath show tiny RPCs associated with slow-wave depolarization [57, 61, 64, 65]. However, these tissues are under tension that opens nonselective cation channels to enhance the influx of Ca^{2+} and release Ca^{2+} from intracellular stores, which then phosphorylate RLC_{20} through the activation of MLCK [66–68].

By contrast, the cardiac muscle cells have a resting membrane potential of about −90 mV. The membrane potential of each depolarization reaches about 20 mV, which causes nearly maximum inward current (I_{max}) for the duration of the plateau potential. This massive calcium influx generates strong contractions with each depolarization to pump blood through the cardiovascular system.

Pharmacomechanical Coupling. The slow wave in gut smooth muscle cells is omnipresent. However, because of subthreshold depolarization at its peak, it is unable, by itself, to generate gut contractions strong enough to mix or propel digesta. However, if the excitatory cholinergic neurons release ACh concurrently with a slow-wave depolarization, the binding of ACh to muscarinic M_3 receptors initiates pharmacomechanical coupling, which activates several intracellular signaling cascades (Figure 11). The seven-transmembrane-spanning M_3 receptors couple to $G\alpha_{q/11}$ protein [69–71]. This G protein couples to nonselective cation channels [72], whose opening allows additional calcium influx, further depolarization of membrane, and phosphorylation of RLC_{20}. The activation of $G\alpha_{q/11}$ also activates phospholipase C (PLC) to hydrolyze phosphatydylinositol biphosphate (PIP_2) and produce diacylglycerol (DAG) and inositol triphosphate (IP_3) [69]. IP_3 acting on its receptors on sarcoplasmic reticulum releases Ca^{2+} from intracellular stores. Together, the increase of intracellular calcium by the three mechanisms depolarizes the membrane beyond mechanical or excitation threshold and prolongs the plateau potential (Figure 12B). The suprathreshold depolarization of smooth muscle membrane induces a series of spikelike depolarizations superimposed on the plateau potential. The peak depolarization of each spike is in the range of 0 to 30 mV, within which the inward current reaches its maximum (I_{max}) (Figure 12A). Each spike induces a short-lived burst of calcium influx. The cumulative calcium from influx and intracellular release enhances MLCK activity and increases RLC_{20} phosphorylation to generate a larger amplitude RPC.

The repolarization of membrane potential, due to inactivation of Ca^{2+} channels and/or opening of Ca^{2+}-activated K^+ channels, terminates the spikes and the contraction. This happens even if the release of ACh continues, which is why enteric neurons and smooth muscle cells together regulate the occurrence of short-duration RPCs.

The pharmacomechanical coupling provides an additional powerful tool to enhance further the amplitude of gut contractions without increasing intracellular calcium concentration. A process called adjustment of calcium sensitivity achieves this [53]. The cell-signaling pathways activated by the binding of ACh to muscarinic M_3 receptors stimulate additional cell-signaling cascades that converge on MLCP to reduce its activity (Figure 11). A decrease in MLCP activity results in net increase of RLC_{20} phosphorylation and hence of contraction amplitude without a change in intracellular calcium concentration. On the other hand, an increase in MLCP activity by the cell-signaling pathways decreases RLC_{20} phosphorylation, without a change in intracellular calcium concentration, and hence decreases the amplitude of smooth muscle contraction.

Figure 11 illustrates a few of these signaling cascades. (1) The activation of protein kinase C (PKC) by diacylglycerol phosphorylates CPI-17, which inhibits PP1c to reduce the activity of MLCP. (2) Arachidonic catalyzed by cPLA$_2$ dissociates MYPT1 and PP1c, thereby reducing the activity of MLCP. (3) The binding of ligands to G$\alpha_{q/11}$/G$_{13}$ converts the inactive form of Rho. GDP to its active form Rho.GTP by Rho-specific guanine exchange factors (RhoGEFs), which activate Rho kinase (ROCK). ROCK phosphorylates MYPT1 to decrease MLCP activity. The decrease in activity by all three signaling pathways increases the phosphorylation of RLC$_{20}$, without a concurrent increase in intracellular concentration.

Figure 11 shows a simplified representation of cell-signaling pathways for pharmacomechanical coupling. Other review articles discuss this topic in depth [52, 53]. These signaling pathways play critical roles in the generation of all three types of colonic contractions, especially GMCs and TCs.

In the human colon, the slow-wave frequency ranges from about 3 to 12 cycles per minute [73–77]; in dogs, it is about 4 to 6 cycles per minute [29]. However, colonic slow waves are highly variable in amplitude and frequency, exhibiting little or no phase locking, which explains the lack of propagation of RPCs in the colon, intensive mixing/turning over, and very slow propulsion (Figure 13A). By contrast, the slow waves in the stomach phase lock and propagate from the corpus to the pylorus (Figure 13B). Note a spike burst after each slow wave during the postprandial period. The slow waves in the duodenum also phase lock (Figure 13C). However, the phase locking of slow waves significantly diminishes in the ileum (Figure 13D).

Some studies propose that the networks of interstitial cells of Cajal (ICCs) regulate the propagation of slow waves [78]. These two-dimensional networks of ICCs are present throughout the gut. However, the slow waves propagate in the stomach and the duodenum but very poorly in the ileum and the colon. Together, these data show that cellular communication across the gap junctions between smooth muscle cells regulates the propagation of slow waves, rather than the ICC networks [79].

According to the above discussion of electromechanical and pharmacomechanical couplings, the maximum frequencies of RPCs cannot exceed their respective slow-wave frequencies. However, in practice, the excitatory cholinergic neurons release ACh in short bursts in response to inputs from the sensory neurons. Therefore, stimulation of pharmacomechanical coupling does not occur during each slow-wave depolarization. In addition, the quantity of ACh release in each burst, which depends on the signals generated by the digesta, is not constant. Therefore, the intensity of pharmacomechanical coupling may differ during each slow-wave depolarization. Taken together, the amplitude and duration of short-duration RPCs vary from one contraction to the next, and their frequency is usually less than the maximum frequency of slow wave. By contrast, the cardiac muscle cells, which depend primarily on electromechanical coupling, contract at the rate of ECG.

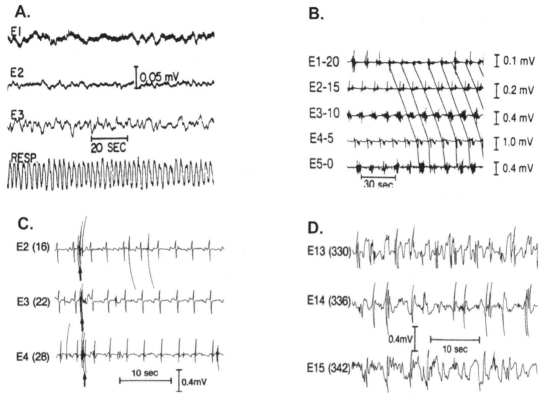

FIGURE 13: The stability and spatial organization of slow waves decreases from the stomach to the colon. (A) Slow waves recorded from the human colon by three electrodes show wide variation in their amplitude from one cycle to the next. The colonic slow waves show no spatial organization (phase locking). Recording electrodes E1 and E2 were 5 cm apart, E2 and E3 3.5 cm apart. (Reproduced with permission from Sarna et al., *Gastroenterology*, 78: 1526–1536, 1980). (B) Gastric slow waves recorded from the canine stomach show regular propagation from the corpus (electrode E-20, 20 cm from the pylorus) to the pylorus (electrode E-0, at the pylorus). Note that a spike burst accompanied each slow wave in the postprandial state during this recording (In in vivo recordings, a sharp biphasic potential corresponds to the upstroke potential in intracellular recordings). (C) Slow waves recorded from the canine duodenum show phase lock, similar to that seen in the stomach. (D) Slow waves recorded from the ileum do not show phase lock. Numbers in parentheses show the distance in cm of recording electrodes (E) from the pylorus. (Reproduced with permission from Sarna, SK, "In vivo myoelectric activity: methods, analysis and interpretation," in *Handbook of Physiology*, eds. Schultz, SG, Wood, JD, and Rauner, BB, *Am Physiol Soc*, Bethesda, MD, 817–863, 1989 [495].)

Take-home Messages

1. A short-duration RPC occurs only if the excitatory cholinergic neurons release ACh during a slow-wave depolarization. The maximum frequency of RPCs at a given site in the gut cannot exceed the frequency of slow waves at that location.
2. The upstroke of slow wave regulates the timing of the start of an RPC.
3. The duration of slow plateau potential determines the maximum duration of RPC.
4. Slow-wave depolarization by itself generates tiny contractions. Concurrent activation of pharmacomechanical coupling by the release of ACh from the cholinergic excitatory motor neurons matures the amplitude of RPCs so that they can perform mixing/turning over and propulsive functions.
5. The slow waves phase lock in the stomach and the duodenum, which facilitate propagation of contractions in these parts of the gut. The phase locking deteriorates distally from there. The colonic slow waves show little or no phase locking. As a result, the RPCs in the colon show little or no propagation, causing mixing and turning over but little propulsion.
6. Intercellular communication across the gap junctions regulates the propagation of slow waves, not the networks of ICCs.

Excitation-Inhibition Coupling. The gut has dual mechanisms to regulate the amplitude, duration, and frequency of smooth muscle contractions. One mechanism, as explained above, is to vary the input to pharmacomechanical coupling by varying the release of ACh. The other is to suppress actively the excitation-contraction coupling in response to signals from the digesta or external sources: CNS, spinal cord, circulating hormones and inflammatory/stress mediators. The inhibitory motor neurons regulate this suppression through the release of NO and VIP, which accumulate, respectively, cyclic guanosine monophosphate (cGMP) and cyclic adenosine monophosphate (cAMP) (Figure 11). The cell signaling initiated by these molecules inhibits smooth muscle contractions by sequestering the intracellular calcium and inhibiting the decrease of MLCP activity [53]. These pathways oppose the effects electromechanical and pharmacomechanical couplings in stimulating contractions in response to the neuronal release of ACh. Significant cross-talk exists between cAMP/protein kinase A (PKA) and cGMP/PKG signaling [53, 80]. At low concentrations, VIP activates PKA exclusively, whereas at higher concentrations, it can cross-activate PKG-I [81–83]. Both kinases inhibit PLC-β1-dependent IP_3 formation by phosphorylation of regulator of G protein signaling (RGS)-4 and accelerating the activation of GTP-bound $G\alpha_{q/11}$ [84]. PKG-I also inhibits IP_3-induced Ca^{2+} release by direct phosphorylation of the sarcoplasmic IP_3 receptors. These kinases can also inhibit cell contraction by Rho A–dependent and Rho A–independent signaling by targeting MYPT1 and CPI-17 [53, 84]. As discussed in the previous section, each of these signaling pathways makes specific contributions to the generation of colonic contractions.

Take-home Message

The activation of inhibitory motor neurons, which release NO and VIP, is an additional means of regulating the amplitude of RPCs.

Cellular Origin and Relaxation Oscillator Characteristics of Slow Waves. The smooth muscle cells communicate with adjacent cells through specialized cell-to-cell junctions, called gap junctions [85]. Their structural and biological characteristics—distances between membranes at the junctions and cylindrical protrusions of one cell membrane into the other—determine the efficacy of communication. Most biological oscillations are of the relaxation oscillator type [86]. The slow-wave oscillations behave as relaxation oscillators; that is, in two electrically coupled cells generating spontaneous oscillations, each cell can modulate the frequency and timing of oscillation of the other cell without altering their intrinsic characteristics. This happens if the frequencies of oscillations of the two cells are not too different from each other [86–89]. In coupled cells, the cell with the higher intrinsic frequency pulls up the lower frequency of the other cell to that of its own, if the electrical coupling between them is strong. The cell with slightly lower intrinsic frequency will begin its depolarization with a short time lag after depolarization of the higher-frequency cell. As a result, the independent oscillations of the two cells, such as slow waves, get phase-locked and show spatial coordination. If the lower-frequency cell is located distal to the higher-frequency cell, as is the case in the gastrointestinal tract, the slow wave propagates in the distal direction. In case of marginal coupling, the cells may entrain part of the time and oscillate independently at their own frequency or at intermediate frequencies the rest of the time. Poor electrical coupling between cells results in the two cells oscillating independently at their own frequencies.

The circular muscle layer in the colon is a few cells thick. However, the upstroke of each slow wave begins almost simultaneously in each cell along the depth of the circular muscle layer at a given location (Figure 14A) [90], which ensures that all cells along the depth of the circular muscle layer contract concurrently to contribute to the strength of the contraction. The simultaneous start of the upstroke potential at various depths of the circular muscle layer shows strong radial coupling of slow waves in this direction, a property of relaxation oscillators. Such coupling in relaxation oscillators does not interfere with the intrinsic characteristics of the oscillators. For example, even though the slow-wave depolarizations are simultaneous, the individual circular muscle cells exhibit a gradient in their resting membrane potential (RMP). The muscle cells closest to the submucosal plexus show most hyperpolarization of RMP, which decreases progressively towards the myenteric

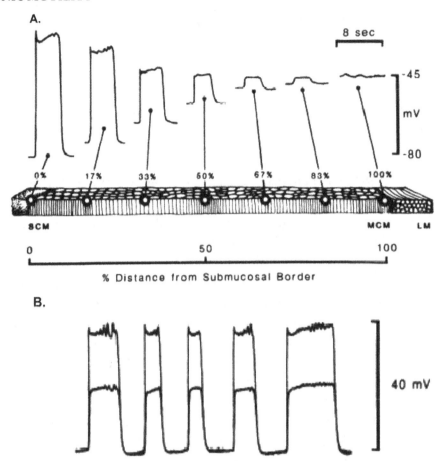

FIGURE 14: (A) Slow waves recorded through the thickness of the circular muscle layer in the canine colon. The slow-wave amplitude is largest in smooth muscle cells close to the submucosal plexus, and it decreases away from this plexus. The RMP of the cells also decreases from the submucosal plexus to the myenteric plexus. The slow waves close to the myenteric plexus are nearly absent and are hard to detect visually. This is because the RMP of the smooth muscle cells close to the myenteric plexus is near the slow-wave reversal potential. (B) The slow waves were synchronous through the thickness of the circular muscle layer. The slow wave of the larger amplitude was from a smooth muscle cell close to the submucosal plexus, while the smaller amplitude slow wave was at the 40% point of thickness. Note that the RMPs at the two locations were aligned. (Reproduced with permission from Smith et al., *Am J Physiol*, 21: C215–C224, 1987 [90].)

plexus (Figure 14B) [57, 90, 91]. The slow-wave characteristics—amplitude, duration and ability to generate spikes—depend strongly on the RMP of the cells [91–94]. Due to the RMP gradient, the amplitude of slow wave decreases progressively from the submucosal plexus to the myenteric plexus (Figure 14B). Of note, the opposite happens in the stomach and the small intestine, which display a negative gradient of RMP in the opposite direction, from the myenteric plexus to the submucosal plexus [92, 95]. We do not know the significance of the differences in the radial morphologies of contractions among different organs. It may relate to differences in the consistencies of the luminal contents in different gut organs.

This specialized radial organization of slow waves is not consistent with the concept that the submucosal interstitial cells of Cajal (ICC-SMs) generate colonic slow waves, which then spread passively (cablelike conduction) through the thickness of the circular muscle layer [78]. The total number of ICC-SM is small (less than 1/25th) when compared with the total number of driven circular muscle cells [96–99]. In particular, the number of ICC-SMs is sparse in the human colon [96, 99], and the ICCs in the human colon make rare gap junctions with other ICCs or to neurons [97]. Therefore, the circular muscle cells would be a large sink for the current generated by the relatively few ICC-SMs.

Colonic slow waves and the short-duration RPCs persist in Ws/Ws rats, which show severe compromise in the presence of all subtypes of ICC [100]. However, the slow waves show less regularity and smaller amplitudes. We do not know whether the instability in slow waves in Ws/Ws rats results from the absence/impairment of ICC or due perturbations in other c-Kit expressing cells, such as mast cells (see review in Ref. [79] for more details).

The separation of the submucosal plexus along with the ICC-SMs from the circular muscle layer depolarizes the RMP of smooth muscle cells closer to the submucosa, thus impairing the RMP gradient [60, 90, 101]. The impairment of RMP reduces slow-wave amplitude and regularity. The precise factor or factors in the submucosal plexus that maintain hyperpolarization of circular smooth muscle cells close to it remain unknown. Carbon monoxide generated by heme oxygenase-1 in the submucosal plexus is a potential candidate for this role [102].

Take-home Messages

1. The slow-wave oscillations behave as relaxation oscillators. This characteristic allows phase locking of slow waves, which is necessary for the propagation of RPCs.
2. The smooth muscle cells generate slow waves. The ICC might play a role in generating the RMP gradient from the submucosal to the myenteric plexus in the colon circular muscle layer.

Regulation of Propagation of Short-Duration RPCs. Figure 15 illustrates the complementary roles of slow waves and enteric neurons in regulating the distance of propagation of short-duration RPCs. Each cell represents a short segment of the colon. In Figure 15A, the adjacent cells couple strongly, and their intrinsic frequencies are close to each other. Therefore, the slow waves are phase locked: the proximal cell depolarizes first, then the middle cell with a short delay, and finally the distal cell with an additional short time lag. As per previous discussions, (1) a short-duration RPC occurs only once during a slow-wave depolarization, (2) its duration is slightly shorter than that of the slow-wave plateau potential, (3) the contraction starts after the upstroke potential, and

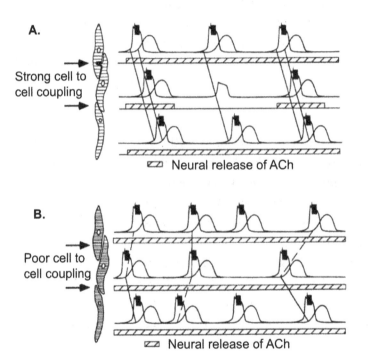

FIGURE 15: Diagram illustrates the complementary roles of slow waves and release of ACh from the excitatory motor neurons in generating propagating and nonpropagating RPCs. (A) The phase lock of the first and third slow waves and concurrent release of ACh (shown by hatched bar) generated propagating contractions. The second slow was also phase locked, but ACh release did not occur at the second cell, resulting in isolated contractions at the proximal and distal cells. (B) The slow waves were not phase locked in this case. The concurrent release of ACh at all three cells resulted in nonpropagating contractions. (Reproduced with permission from Sarna, SK. "Myoelectric and Contractile Activities of the Gastrointestinal Tract," in *Schuster Atlas of Gastrointestinal Motility*, 2nd ed., eds. Schuster, MM, Crowell, MD, and Koch, KL, BD Decker Inc. Hamilton and London, 1–18, 2002 [496].)

(4) finally, this contraction occurs only if the excitatory motor neurons release ACh during depolarization. In the case of the first propagating slow wave, ACh release occurred concurrently at each of the three segments represented by these cells. Therefore, the contraction occurred first in the proximal segment, then at the middle and distal segments with the same time lags as the slow wave. Consequently, the contraction propagated from the proximal to the distal segment.

During the second slow wave, the excitatory motor neurons release ACh only in the first and the third segments during their slow-wave depolarizations. In this case, the contraction did not propagate from the first to the third segment but instead occurred independently in the first and the third segments. However, the third slow wave had concurrent release of ACh in all three segments, and the third contraction propagated, like the first.

Figure 15B shows a case where the electrical coupling between adjacent cells is poor. Therefore, the slow waves in adjacent cells are not phase locked; they occur independently. In this situation, even if the excitatory motor neurons release ACh concurrently over the entire length of the three segments, the contractions will not propagate, because each contraction during a slow-wave depolarization starts shortly after its upstroke potential. The contractions in each segment will follow the spatial discoordination of slow waves.

In essence, the slow waves alone regulate the timing and direction of propagation of short-duration RPCs. The excitatory motor neurons regulate whether or not the short-duration RPCs will occur. As discussed earlier, this function of the excitatory motor neurons is modifiable by the inhibitory motor neurons. Finally, the slow waves and excitatory motor neurons together regulate the frequency and distance of propagation of each short-duration RPC. A short-duration RPC will propagate only up to the distance over which the slow waves are phase locked. Even when slow waves are phase locked, a short-duration RPC will propagate only over the length of the gut segment over which the excitatory motor neurons concurrently release ACh.

Take-home Message
Phase lock of slow waves and the concurrent release of ACh together regulate the direction and distance of propagation of RPCs.

Types of Enteric Neurons and Their Functional Significance. Enteric neurons are classified according to function, morphology, electrophysiological characteristics, and chemical coding [49, 103–106, 106a]. Functional classification identifies three types of neurons: (1) motor neurons, (2) interneurons, and (3) intrinsic sensory neurons (ISNs). Morphologically, the vast majority of enteric neurons are of two types, Dogiel type I and Dogiel type II [107]. Type I neurons are monoaxonal with lamellar dendrites (Figure 15A). Dogiel type II neurons are multiaxonal with or without dendrites (Figure 15B). Type I neurons have a narrow field of influence while type II neurons have a broader field of influence because of their multiaxonal structure. Therefore, type II neurons can integrate information from a larger field and, in turn, send the effector signal over a broad field. Consequently, these neurons are best suited to sense the characteristics of digesta at several adjacent locations in the lumen and coordinate the motor response to generate a circumferential contraction over a short segment of the colon.

By electrophysiological characteristics, the neurons are classified as S–type I and AH (after hyperpolarization)–type II. Both types of neurons generate slow excitatory postsynaptic potentials (sEPSPs) and fast EPSPs (fEPSPs) (Figure 16). A fast EPSP lasts from a few milliseconds to a few seconds (Figure 16A). It usually associates with a single action potential or a brief burst of action potentials. The conduction of these action potentials over an axon or a dendrite depolarizes them to induce calcium influx and release neurotransmitters. Accordingly, each fast EPSP releases a small quantity of neurotransmitter for a short time. By contrast, the depolarization during a slow EPSP lasts from about 10 to 60 seconds [108, 109]. Consequently, a slow EPSP may induce a long series of action potentials resulting in almost continuous release of neurotransmitters for the duration of the train of action potentials (Figure 16B). The result is an accumulation of the neurotransmitter at the neuroeffector junction.

In AH–type II neurons, brief hyperpolarization follows each action potential [103] (Figure 16C). The functional significance after hyperpolarization is to prevent the immediate generation of another sEPSP, which allows time for regeneration/mobilization of neurotransmitters for the next release. Note that fast EPSPs may not require hyperpolarization because they are of short duration with a limited number of action potentials.

Motor Neurons. Two types of motor neurons project from the myenteric plexus to the circular muscle layer: the excitatory motor neurons and the inhibitory motor neurons (Figure 10). These are Dogiel type I monoaxonal neurons with a narrow field of influence. However, the axons of the motor neurons branch extensively along the circumference within the circular muscle layer to broaden their field of influence in this direction [110, 111] (Figure 16A). This configuration facilitates the concurrent release of neurotransmitter around the circumference, resulting in a ringlike contraction.

The excitatory and inhibitory inputs to the smooth muscle cells act like the accelerator and the braking system of an automobile, respectively. In the resting state, low-level release of excitatory and inhibitory neurotransmitters counterbalance each other to maintain resting tone. As discussed in the section on excitation-contraction coupling, additional release of ACh from the cholinergic excitatory neurons overwhelms the low-level inhibitory input, and the cells contract. This is equivalent to stepping on the accelerator of an automobile. However, if there is also a concurrent increase in the release of an inhibitory neurotransmitter, the excitation-inhibition coupling gener-

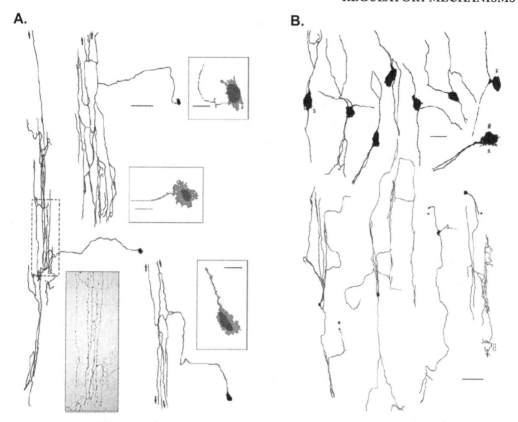

FIGURE 16: Morphologies of Dogiel type I and type II neurons. (A) Three examples of Dogiel type I circular muscle motor neurons. Images of the cell bodies are shown at high power; the projections are at a lower power. The axons branch out to promote a circumferentially oriented plexus in the circular muscle. Some axons projected farther than shown above. Insert shows photomicrograph of part of the circular muscle innervation (boxed area). Scale bar = 20 µm in inserts. (B) Morphologies of Dogiel type II neurons injected with biotin. Cells were drawn with the aid of a camera lucida. The nerve cells were round or oval with generally smooth surface and long projections. Long processes tended to run in circular direction (vertical in the figure). Asterisks indicate expansion bulbs where processes were broken off during initial dissection. Scale bar at top 50 µm for the uppermost eight neurons, the bottom bar 100 µm for four lower neurons. (Reproduced with permission from Nurgali et al. and Furmess, JB, *J Comp Neurol*, 468: 112–124, 2004 [146].)

ated by it partially or completely overcomes the excitation-contraction coupling and suppresses the contractions or blocks them completely. Evidence for concurrent excitatory and inhibitory inputs to smooth muscle cells comes from findings that in vivo administration of the nNOS inhibitor L-NAME enhances the amplitudes of RPCs in fasting as well as the postprandial state [112, 113, 113a]. The concurrent excitatory and inhibitory inputs to smooth muscle cells is a mechanism that varies randomly the amplitudes of RPCs for effective mixing and turning over of luminal contents as well as varying the distance of their propagation (see section on regulation of propagation of RPCs). The excitation-inhibition coupling in circular smooth muscle cells is critical in producing descending inhibition of contractions ahead of a GMC [9, 114–116].

The mapping of excitatory and inhibitory motor neurons from the myenteric plexus to the circular muscle layer with DiI shows that they project proximally or distally an average of about 2 mm [117]. The majority of ChAT-containing excitatory neurons project orally from the cell body, and the nNOS-containing inhibitory motor neurons project anally. It has been suggested that these polarized projections facilitate ascending excitatory and descending inhibitory reflexes. However, an average colonic RPC occupies about 10 mm of the colon while a GMC occupies a 20- to 30-cm segment. It is, therefore, unlikely that oral or anal projections of the motor neurons over a few millimeters would materially contribute to the ascending and inhibitory reflexes. The motor neurons communicate primarily with smooth muscle cells located in the same plane. Oral and aboral communication occurs primarily via interneurons that project more than 10 mm in each direction and can relay signals over several ganglia.

Some studies have proposed that intramuscular interstitial cells of Cajal (ICC-IMs) serve as obligatory intermediaries between the motor neurons and smooth muscle cells [118–120]. The concept is that the excitatory and inhibitory neurotransmitters of the motor neurons excite the ICC-IM, which then project a composite signal to the smooth muscle cells to contract or not. The nature of this composite signal is unknown [79]. *This concept invokes wired neuromuscular transmission at the gap junctions between the nerve varicosities and circular smooth muscle cells [79]* (Figure 17). However, the smooth muscle cells vastly outnumber the ICC-IM. This kind of neuromuscular communication will not stimulate all smooth muscle cells in the neighborhood to contract concurrently; in fact, under this scheme, most circular smooth muscle cells will never receive an ICC or neuronal input. More importantly, the activation of pharmacomechanical coupling in smooth muscle cells is essential to generate contractions that can mix/turn over and propel luminal contents (see section on excitation-contraction coupling). The ICCs are nonneuronal cells; they do not synthesize ACh and therefore cannot induce pharmacomechanical coupling in smooth muscle cells. Accumulating electrophysiological, immunohistochemical, and morphological evidence shows that the smooth muscle cells and ICC-IM independently receive neuronal inputs [121–126]. The ICC do not serve as intermediaries between the enteric motor neurons and smooth muscle cells [79, 127, 128]. *The*

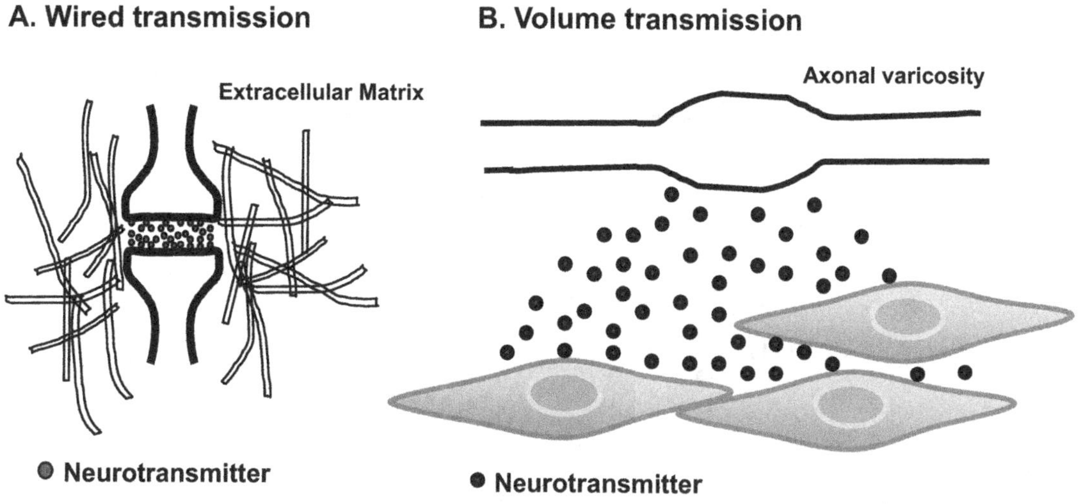

A. Wired transmission

Extracellular Matrix

● **Neurotransmitter**

B. Volume transmission

Axonal varicosity

● **Neurotransmitter**

FIGURE 17: Diagrams illustrate differences between wired and volume transmissions between neurons and effector cells. (A) Wired transmission is 1:1 between neurons and effector cells. (B) In volume transmission, the neurotransmitter diffuses in the extracellular medium to affect multiple cells in the neighborhood. (Reproduced with permission from Sarna, SK, *Am J Physiol Gastrointest Liver Physiol*, 294: 372–390, 2008 [79].)

motor neurons communicate directly with the smooth muscle cells by volume transmission, in which the neurotransmitter released from the varicosities of multiple fibers accumulates in the extracellular medium to concurrently affect a large volume of effector cells [129–132] (Figure 18).

Interneurons. The interneurons in the colon are largely Dogiel type I [133]. These interneurons project more than 10 mm in the oral, anal, and circumferential directions to communicate signals among adjacent ganglia [110]. The descending projections of interneurons outnumber the ascending projections by a ratio of 4:1 [110]. The interneurons may synapse on excitatory and inhibitory motor neurons in the target ganglia to stimulate the release of their respective neurotransmitters, or they may synapse on other interneurons to form a relay system that projects the signal over longer distances (Figure 19).

About 90% of the ascending interneurons and about 50% of descending interneurons contain ChAT alone or ChAT with nNOS. In both cases, the cholinergic interneurons synapse on nicotinic receptors. Consequently, hexamethonium blocks oral/anal transmission as well as the stimulation of motor neurons in the lateral direction [47, 134, 135]. The ascending and descending cholinergic interneurons that synapse on inhibitory motor neurons produce ascending and descending

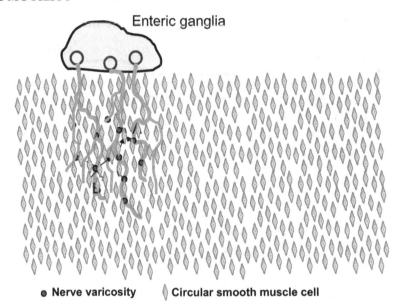

Enteric ganglia

● **Nerve varicosity**   ◊ **Circular smooth muscle cell**

FIGURE 18: In volume transmission, each circular muscle cell concurrently receives neurotransmitters from several varicosities, and each varicosity supplies neurotransmitters to several smooth muscle cells. (Reproduced with permission from Sarna, SK, *Am J Physiol Gastrointest Liver Physiol*, 294: 372–390, 2008 [79].)

inhibition of contractions, respectively, and those that synapse on cholinergic excitatory motor neurons produce ascending or descending stimulation of contractions (Figure 19).

A small number of descending interneurons in the colon are also immunoreactive for VIP, tachykinins, 5-HT, neuropeptide Y, galanin, somatostatin, and met-encephalin [136–139]. However, the precise roles of these neurotransmitters as well as of NO in interneurons remain unknown.

Intrinsic Sensory Neurons. The cell bodies of ISNs are located in the submucosal and myenteric ganglia with axonal endings in the mucosa, muscle layers, and muscularis submucosa to detect the presence of digesta and its chemical nature, as well as wall tension due to a contraction or distension of the colon wall [104, 140–143]. These neurons transmit sensory information directly to the motor neurons in the same plane or indirectly through a chain of interneurons to motor neurons of ganglia oral or aboral to the plane of ISN.

Most ISNs are of the multiaxonal Dogiel type II/AH [110, 144–148]. In response to a chemical or mechanical stimulus from the lumen or within the gut wall, they transmit the signal to their large field of influence, which results in a ringlike contraction over an appreciable length of the

B.

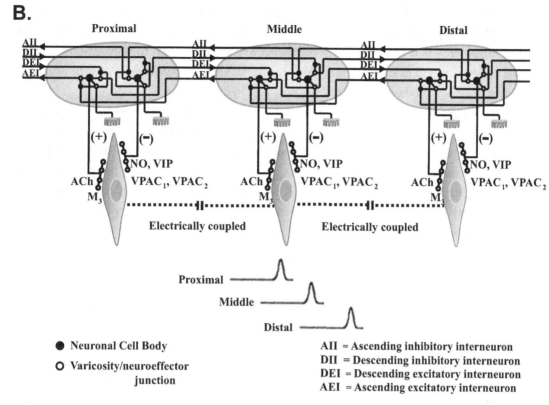

FIGURE 19: Schematic diagram provides an overview of the ascending and descending communication among ganglia in the myenteric plexus. The interneurons project orally and anally. They synapse on both the excitatory and inhibitory motor neurons in oral and anal directions to provide ascending excitation and inhibition as well as descending excitation and inhibition. The interneurons also synapse on other interneurons to transmit the signal to the next ganglion in the chain. The interneurons also project in the circumferential direction (not shown here). The neurotransmitter of excitatory motor neurons is ACh, and of inhibitory motor neurons, NO and VIP. The binding of ACh to muscarinic M_3 receptor on smooth muscle cells initiates excitation-contraction coupling in the cells. The smooth muscle cell contracts when there is a net increase in the phosphorylation of RLC_{20}. For RPCs, the slow wave in circular smooth muscle cells regulates the timing and frequency of contractions at each location. See Figures 10 and 11 for additional details.

colon segment (~1 cm for RPC). In the guinea pig small intestine, mucosal stimuli evoke both fast and slow EPSPs in postsynaptic neurons [142]. Tetrodotoxin, hexamethonium, ω-conotoxin, and low Ca^{2+}/high mg^{2+}- in the medium block the fast EPSPs, indicating that their generation requires neuronal conduction and at least one nicotinic synapse. CGRP antagonists—but not nicotinic receptor antagonist hexamethonium—block the slow EPSPs in ISNs.

Most of the gut, including the colon, generates spontaneous contractions in the absence of any digesta in the lumen [149]. The neuronal input for these contractions comes from enteric neurons (both Dogiel types I and II) that generate spontaneous fast EPSPs and slow EPSPs [110] (Figure 10). These neurons release neurotransmitters at the neuroeffector junction through the motor neurons. Several types of neurons generate spontaneous rhythmic or arrhythmic activity [150–152]. Rhythmic activity of the enteric neurons generates the cyclic migrating motor complexes in the interdigestive state [135, 153].

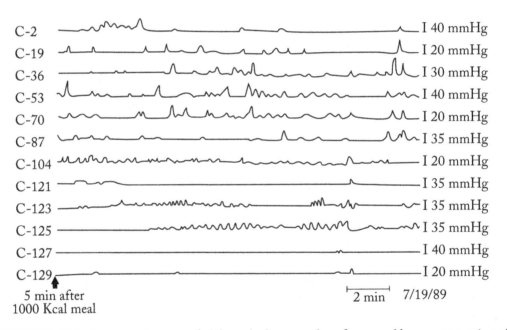

FIGURE 20: Colonic contractions recorded from the human colon after a meal by a manometric catheter. The RPCs are disorganized in time and space, as shown in Figure 1C. The tip of the manometric catheter rested near the cecum. The numbers after C indicate the distances in cm of the side openings in the manometric tube from the tip of the manometric tube. (Reproduced with permission from Sarna, SK, and Shi, Xuan-Zheng. *Physiology of the Gastrointestinal Tract*, 4th ed., Vol. 1, eds. Johnson, LR, Barrett, KE, Merchant, JL, Gishan, FK, Said, HM, and Wood, JD, Chapter 39, 965–993, 2006.)

The timing of slow waves in smooth muscle cells is independent of the generation of EPSPs. Therefore, the release of an excitatory or inhibitory neurotransmitter may not exactly coincide with the slow-wave depolarization. A partial overlap between slow-wave depolarization and a fast EPSP means a smaller number of action potentials during a plateau potential than if the same fast EPSP had completely overlapped with the plateau potential. This is one of the reasons that the amplitude of postprandial contractions varies from one contraction to the next and all RPCs do not propagate, even if the slow waves are phase locked (Figure 20).

Take-home Message

1. The ICC-IMs do not act as intermediaries between the motor neurons and smooth muscle cells; the motor neurons innervate the smooth muscle cells directly to contract them.
2. Spontaneously active enteric neurons provide the input for smooth muscle cells to contract in the absence of digesta in the lumen.
3. ACh and NO are the primary physiological neurotransmitters of excitatory and inhibitory motor neurons. Substance P and VIP may serve these roles in special situations.
4. The interneurons, rather than the very short distances of oral and anal projections of motor neurons, mediate the oral and anal communication in the gut.

Long-Duration RPCs

The colon is unique in the gastrointestinal tract in generating the short-duration (discussed above) and long-duration RPCs [29, 30]. The duration of long-duration RPCs is several-fold longer than that of a slow-wave depolarization. Therefore, the slow-wave depolarizations do not regulate the long-duration RPCs. Instead, the colonic circular smooth muscle cells spontaneously but, intermittently, generate high amplitude depolarizations at a frequency of about 25 to 40 cycles per minute, called contractile electrical complex [29, 30] (Figure 21). Spikes occur during each depolarization of the contractile electrical complex (Figure 21). Each spike burst results in a strong contraction regulated by electromechanical and pharmacomechanical couplings similar to those described for short-duration RPCs (Figure 11). However, because of the high frequency of depolarizations in a contractile electrical complex, the individual spikes nearly fuse to become a long-duration spike burst and, thus, a long-duration contraction [29, 30, 154] (Figure 21). The duration of these contractions depends on the duration of the contractile electrical complex [29]. In vitro experiments with circular muscle strips devoid of the myenteric and submucosal plexi show that higher concentrations of $BaCl_2$ and Bay K 8644 generate high-frequency depolarizations in a contractile electrical complex [155]. We know very little about cell signaling for the generation of long-duration RPCs.

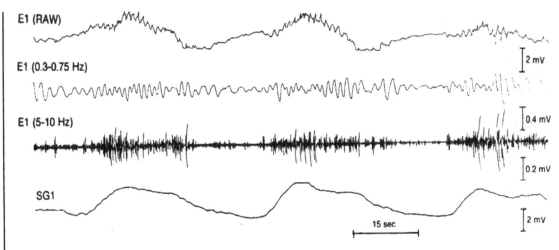

FIGURE 21: Contractile electrical complexes generate long-duration RPCs in the colon. A combined strain gauge transducer and bipolar electrode recorded contractions and electrical activity concurrently from the same location in the canine colon. The top tracing shows three incidents of contractile electrical complexes. The second tracing from the top shows the electrical tracing filtered to show the oscillations at 25 to 40 cycles per minute in each complex. The next tracing shows an almost continuous burst of spikes in filtered electrical activity, whose duration was the same as that of the corresponding contractile electrical complex. The bottom tracing shows long-duration contractions generated by each contractile electrical complex. (Reproduced with permission from Sarna, SK, *Am J Physiol Gastrointest Liver Physiol*,13: G213–G220, 1986 [29].)

Take-home Messages

1. Spontaneous oscillations of smooth muscle cells called contractile electrical complexes regulate the occurrence of long-duration RPCs in the colon.
2. The slow waves are omnipresent; the contractile electrical complexes are not.
3. The contractile electrical complexes propagate over longer distances than the slow waves.

GIANT MIGRATING CONTRACTIONS

The duration of a GMC is several-fold longer than that of a slow wave. Therefore, the slow waves cannot regulate GMCs. Our understanding of the cellular mechanisms of stimulation of GMCs is limited because ex vivo tissues of nonrodent species do not generate GMCs. However, experiments by close intra-arterial infusions in conscious animals have provided some insights. Of note is the finding that, in the canine ileum, close arterial infusion of CGRP, one of the neurotransmitter of

ISNs [156], stimulates RPCs at smaller concentrations and GMCs at higher concentrations [116]. The inhibition of nicotinic receptors by hexamethonium or inhibition of muscarinic receptors by atropine blocks both RPCs and GMCs. Therefore, CGRP acts on presynaptic neurons, requiring a nicotinic synapse to stimulate the release of ACh from motor neurons at the neuromuscular junction. By contrast, close intra-arterial infusions of several other neurotransmitters/agonists—serotonin, ACh, erythromycin, and motilin—stimulate only RPCs [45, 157].

Electrophysiological findings show that CGRP stimulates both fast and slow EPSPs [108, 109]. Presumably, low doses of CGRP stimulate fast EPSPs to stimulate a short burst of ACh release at the neuromuscular junction, generating RPCs. Higher doses of CGRP stimulate slow EPSPs to stimulate a prolonged burst of ACh release, resulting in its accumulation at the neuromuscular junction and generation of GMCs (Figure 22). Experiments with close intra-arterial infusion of neostigmine, a cholinesterase inhibitor, confirm this hypothesis by showing that the accumulation of ACh at the neuromuscular junction stimulates GMCs [134].

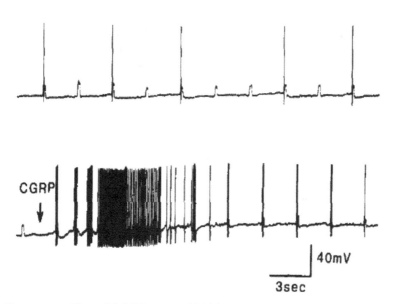

FIGURE 22: Excitatory effect of CGRP on an AH/Type II myenteric neuron. Top and bottom tracings are continuous. Constant current depolarizing pulses were injected repetitively into the cell. The cell either did not discharge action potentials to depolarizing pulses or fired a single action potential followed by a long-lasting hyperpolarizing afterpotential prior to a 20 msec pulse of 20 μM CGRP, shown by arrow. Application of CGRP evoked membrane depolarization, repetitive action potential discharges to depolarizing pulses, and the occurrence of spontaneous action potentials. (Reproduced with permission from Palmer et al. and Wood, JD, *European Journal of Pharmacology*, 132: 163–170, 1986 [109].)

The sustained release of ACh at the neuromuscular junction activates $G\alpha_q$, which opens $Ca_v1.2b$ (L-type) calcium channels. The influx of calcium depolarizes the cell membrane beyond the excitation threshold, inducing a long train of spikes [158, 159] (Figure 23), which causes additional calcium influx. This calcium influx is critical to initiating a GMC because L-type calcium channel blockers verapamil or nifedipine block this depolarization as well as the spikes and the GMC associated with them [12, 16, 116, 160, 161]. The pharmacomechanical coupling activated

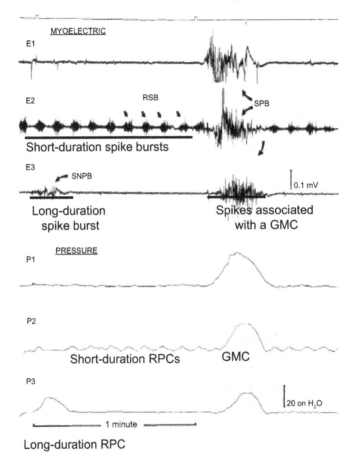

FIGURE 23: Myoelectric correlates of GMCs and RPCs in the human sigmoid colon recorded with a manometric catheter combined with ring-type electrodes. The three recording sites were 15 cm apart. The top three tracings show myoelectric activity; the bottom three show contractile activity. Each short-spike burst was associated with an RPC. The long-spike bursts were associated with a long-duration RPC. None of the RPCs propagated. Longer and stronger spike bursts were associated with a GMC that propagated from the first recording site to the last. (Reproduced with permission from Schang et al., *Dig Dis and Sciences*, 12: 1331–1337, 1986 [158].)

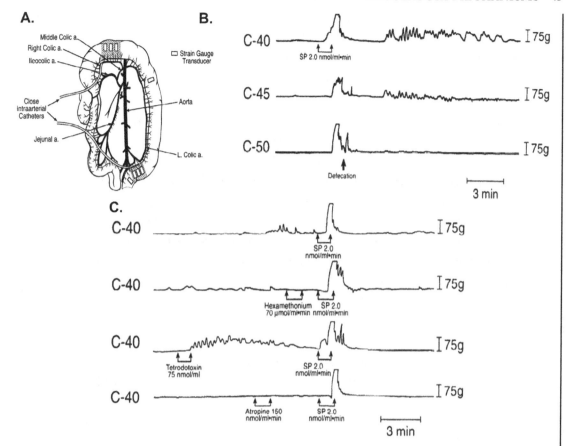

FIGURE 24: Close intra-arterial infusion of substance P in the canine colon stimulates GMCs at the higher infusion rate of 2 nmol/ml/min for 1 minute. (A) Diagram shows the placement of an intra-arterial catheter to infuse selectively small doses of substance P in a local segment. Similar intravenous infusions of substance P have no effect. (B) Substance P infusion stimulated a GMC that propagated distally, resulting in defecation. (C) Prior infusions of hexamethonium to block nicotinic receptors, tetrodotoxin to block enteric neuronal conduction of action potentials, and atropine to block muscarinic receptors had no effect on the stimulation of GMCs by substance P. C = colonic strain gauge transducer. The numbers after C indicate the distance in cm of the transducers from the ileocolonic junction. (Reproduced with permission from Tsukamoto et al. and Sarna, SK, *Am J Physiol Gastrointest Liver Physiol*, 35: G1607–G1614, 1997 [163].)

by high concentrations of ACh utilizes different cell signaling pathways than those activated by lower concentrations [116, 162, 163, 164].

Low doses of substance P stimulate colonic RPCs, whereas higher doses stimulate both GMCs and RPCs. Tetrodotoxin that blocks the conduction of action potentials and atropine reduce RPCs by about half, indicating that substance P acts concurrently on motor neurons to release ACh and on smooth muscle cells to stimulate RPCs. However, tetrodotoxin, atropine, or hexamethonium do not block the stimulation of GMCs by the higher doses of substance P, indicating a direct effect on smooth muscle cells [163]. Interestingly, the response to NK1 agonist decreases in the inflamed colon, whereas the sensitivity of substance P to stimulate GMCs increases. It is noteworthy that colonic inflammation suppresses the RPCs and, at the same time, enhances the generation of GMCs [165, 166]. These bimodal effects of inflammation are responsible for diarrhea in colonic inflammation. The above findings suggest that the opposite effects of inflammation on colonic motor function are due to the utilization of different signaling pathways of excitation-contraction coupling in smooth muscle cells [167].

Take-home Messages

1. Slow waves do not regulate the generation of GMCs.
2. A long-duration release of ACh and its accumulation at the neuromuscular junction stimulates a GMC.
3. Slow EPSPs generating a long train of action potentials release copious amounts of ACh to stimulate a GMC.
4. The cell-signaling pathways of pharmacomechanical coupling to generate GMCs differ from those that generate RPCs.
5. Substance P acting directly on smooth muscle cells is one of the mediators for the generation of colonic GMCs.

TONIC CONTRACTIONS

The stimulation of $G\alpha_{q/11}$ coupled receptors in smooth muscle cells also activates Rho A (GTP. Rho A), a small (20-kDa) monomeric GTPase [168]. Rho is retained in the cytoplasm in its inactive form GDP.Rho A in the resting state of smooth muscle cells (Figure 11). The activation of Rho A is catalyzed by guanine nucleotide exchange factors (GEFs) to exchange GTP for GDP, translocating it to the membrane where it binds to the regulatory binding domain of serine/threonine Rho kinase (ROK) to autophosphorylate it through a conformational change [53, 169, 170]. The activated ROK phosphorylates MYPT1 at Thr-696, reducing the dephosphorylation rate of

RLC_{20} and thereby enhancing Ca^{2+}-sensitivity (Figure 11). ROK mediates slow tonic contraction in vascular smooth muscle cells; we do not know its role in increasing tone in colonic smooth muscle cells. However, ROK and PKC mediate the sustained contraction in rabbit gastric smooth muscle cells [84, 171, 172]. The tonic contractions mediated by ROK-induced phosphorylation of MYPT1 occurs under low $[Ca^{2+}]_i$ conditions. The low-level increase in $[Ca^{2+}]_i$ produced by Ca^{2+} influx may be required to phosphorylate RLC_{20}, as this contraction in vivo is blocked also by the inhibition of $Ca_v1.2$ channels. Slow waves do not regulate tonic contractions; pharmacomechanical coupling activated by ACh alone generates tone.

Take-home Messages

1. Slow waves do not regulate tonic contractions.
2. The cell-signaling pathways of pharmacomechanical coupling to generate tone are different from those that generate GMCs or RPCs.
3. Table 1 shows which regulatory mechanisms contribute to the generation of the three types of contractions: RPCs, GMCs, and TCs.

EXCITATION-TRANSCRIPTION COUPLING

Recent findings show that enteric neurons do more than just work with smooth muscle cells to regulate different types of gut contractions. A continuous low-level release of neurotransmitters, such as VIP, induces transcription of the cell-signaling proteins of excitation-contraction coupling in smooth muscle cells [173]. One of the targets of VIP is *Cacna1C* gene encoding the pore-forming α_{1C} subunit of $Ca_v1.2b$ (L-type) calcium channels. The incubation of primary cultures of human colon circular smooth muscle cells with VIP time- and concentration-dependently enhances transcription of the *Cacna1c* gene, resulting in an increase in the number of calcium channel pores in smooth muscle membrane (Figure 25). As a result, the net amount of calcium reflux increases in response to the same quantity of ACh released, enhancing the contractile response. Systemic administration of VIP in rats for seven days by an osmotic pump also enhances expression of the α_{1C}-subunit, resulting in increase reactivity to ACh, faster colonic transit, and an increased defecation rate [174]. The systemic administration of VIP receptor antagonists has opposite effects.

These findings show that the expression of cell-signaling proteins is plastic and can be altered by changes in their microenvironment [62, 175–177]. Such plasticity may explain motility dysfunctions as well as presenting targets to developing therapeutic agents to treat motility disorders [174].

TABLE 1: Contributions of core regulating mechanisms to the spatiotemporal characteristics of different types of gut contractions

	RHYTHMIC PHASIC CONTRACTIONS					TONE	ULTRAPROPULSIVE CONTRACTIONS	
	FREQUENCY	AMPLITUDE	DURATION	DIRECTION OF PROPAGATION	DISTANCE OF PROPAGATION	AMPLITUDE	AMPLITUDE	DIRECTION OF PROPAGATION
Slow waves	×	×	×	×	×	–	–	–
Enteric neurons	×	×	×	–	×	×	×	×
Excitation-contraction and excitation-inhibition couplings	×	×	×	–	–	×	×	–

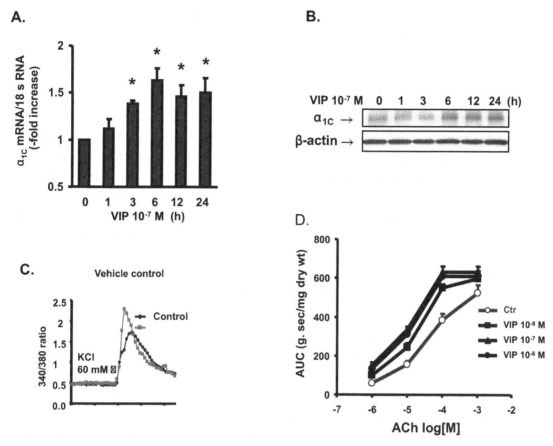

FIGURE 25: Low concentrations of VIP induce gene expression of the α_{1C} subunit of $Ca_v1.2$ (L-type) calcium channels to enhance motility function. (A and B) Incubation of primary cultures of human colonic circular smooth muscle cells with VIP enhanced mRNA and protein expression of the α_{1C} subunit of $Ca_v1.2$ (L-type) calcium channels. (C) KCl-induced calcium influx was greater in colonic smooth muscle cells incubated with VIP for 24 hours, as compared with that in those incubated with control medium. (D) The incubation of human colonic circular smooth muscle strips with VIP enhanced their reactivity to ACh.

Take-home Messages

1. Low-level spontaneous release of VIP induces expression of the *Cacna1c* gene that encodes the α_{1C}-subunit of $Ca_v1.2b$ (L-type) calcium channels.
2. The expression of cell-signaling proteins is plastic. Alterations in their expression may underlie motility disorders.

3. Therapeutic agents that adjust the expression of cell-signaling proteins may normalize motility function in disease.

ENTERIC REFLEXES

A reflex is an involuntary movement in response to a stimulus. In the gut, the reflex may be excitatory (smooth muscle contracts in response to a change in luminal contents or distension/compression of gut wall) or inhibitory (suppression of ongoing smooth muscle contractions by a change in luminal contents or compression/distension of gut wall). These reflexes can be short, in which the response occurs at the site of the stimulus or close to it. In long reflexes, the response occurs in a gut organ different from the one that generates the stimulus, or it may occur at a distant location in the same organ. In general, enteric neurons and autonomic nerves, respectively, mediate short and long reflexes.

As shown in Figure 19, interneurons relay signals between the adjacent ganglia in oral, anal, and circumferential directions. The interneurons projecting in the ascending or descending direction synapse on excitatory and inhibitory motor neurons that project into the thickness of the circular muscle layer. Therefore, interneurons can stimulate or inhibit contractions oral to the site of the stimulus if they are ascending excitatory and inhibitory reflexes, respectively. Likewise, interneurons projecting in the descending direction can stimulate or inhibit contractions in a gut segment anal to the stimulus if they are descending excitatory and inhibitory reflexes, respectively.

Of all types of possible enteric reflexes, the one that putatively stimulates contractions above the site of stimulation and simultaneously inhibits contractions/relaxes tone below it (peristaltic reflex) has received the most attention. Bayliss and Starling [24] first noted this reflex in the canine small intestine. Their experiments were imaginative and innovative for science at the end of the 19th century. However, their experiments were fraught with confounding factors arising from the experimental preparation (castor oil cleansing; morphine analgesia; immersion of whole animal, except head, in warm saline solution) and experimental methods (use of inflated balloon to record intestinal contractions and relaxations, use of a lump of cotton wool of unspecified size coated with Vaseline/soap, or using pinch as stimulus). They made only visual observations of oral contractions propelling the bolus. It is not clear whether a single contraction or a series of contractions induced descending inhibition. However, the duration of descending inhibition was several-fold longer than the duration of an oral rhythmic contraction.

The lack of physiological conditions in their experiments is acceptable due to the limited knowledge in that era. However, one wonders whether they would have noted stimulation of ascending contractions and descending inhibition in canine small intestine under more physiological conditions and with appropriate recording methods. Regardless, Bayliss and Starling proclaimed the peristaltic reflex of ascending contraction and descending inhibition as the basis of propulsion in the gut. However, several investigators in the first half of the 20th century could not reproduce their findings and challenged the law of the intestine [178–181]. If propulsion in the gut were to occur by stereotypic reflexes, digesta will move at the same rate throughout its length. This does not happen.

In spite of the limitations of Bayliss and Starling's study and doubts about the interpretation of their data, the seminal findings that intraluminal stimulation transmits a bidirectional neural signal to the smooth muscle cells took hold. Several decades of research on this topic, using electrophysiological, immunohistochemical, and organ bath approaches in flat sheets of colon or small intestine and ex-vivo segments, mostly from rodents and guinea pigs, have firmly established the following [50, 51, 114, 115, 144, 147, 182–187].

1. Focal stimulation of the mucosa or circumferential stretch simultaneously transmits an excitatory signal to a limited length in the oral direction and an inhibitory signal in the anal direction.
2. This transmission occurs via nicotinic synapses in interneurons.
3. The signal in the oral direction releases ACh from the excitatory motor neurons at smaller intensities of stimulation and substance P at higher stimulation intensities.
4. Depending on the type of preparation and the animal species, the excitatory neurotransmitters stimulate an excitatory junctional potential (EJP) in circular smooth muscle cells, increase the tone of circular smooth muscle cells, or stimulate RPCs, whose intensity depends on the intensity of the stimulus.
5. The signal in the anal direction releases NO and VIP in the descending segment, generating an inhibitory junction potential in smooth muscle cells (IJP) and relaxing their tone.
6. Mucosal stroking or circumferential stretch releases 5-HT from enterochromafin (EC) cells in the affected area of the circular muscle strip.
7. 5-HT stimulates 5-HT$_{1P}$/5-HT$_4$ receptors on ISN nerve endings in the mucosa, which releases CGRP/ACh to stimulate simultaneously the oral and anal projecting interneurons in the area of their influence [182, 184, 188].
8. Additional 5-HT$_4$ receptors on ISN nerve endings may modulate the release of ACh and CGRP from the ISNs [142].

These elegant studies have greatly advanced our understanding of the morphology of lumen-to-myenteric-plexus signals in response to focal mucosal stimulation or by circumferential distension. However, the concurrent release of excitatory neurotransmitters in an oral segment and that of inhibitory neurotransmitters in an anal segment is just the first in a series of steps that result in

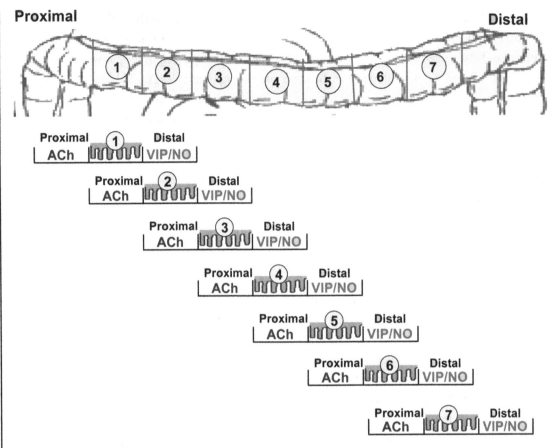

FIGURE 26: Ascending excitation and descending inhibition in response to concurrent focal stimulation of mucosa by digesta at multiple locations releases both ACh and NO/VIP at all locations. The circular smooth muscle cells in segment 2 receive ACh due to ascending excitation from segment 3. At the same time, the cells in this segment receive NO/VIP due to descending inhibition from mucosal stimulation in segment 1. The net amplitude of contractions in segment 2 depends on the relative intensity of excitation-contraction and excitation-inhibition couplings stimulated by ACh and NO/VIP, respectively. The ascending excitation and descending inhibition by itself does not cause propulsion, which occurs only when the RPCs propagate due to the coordinated actions of the release of these neurotransmitters and phase-locked slow waves. Note that, in the colon, the slow waves show very poor phase lock.

mixing/turning over or propulsion of digesta. *This reflex by itself does not propel any digesta.* The propulsion in the gut does not occur by generating a higher pressure at one location, as in the cardiovascular system. Propulsion occurs by propagating contractions, for which slow waves and excitation-contraction coupling must participate. For example, the above reflex occurs almost everywhere in the colon all the time due to the presence of fecal material. However, the slow waves do not phase lock, so that RPCs in the colon do not usually propagate and cause very little propulsion. More importantly, the RPCs do not compress the colon wall strongly enough to produce descending inhibition. Only GMCs do this (Figure 4).

In real life, there is no single-point stimulation of mucosa or circumferential stretch in a short segment of the gut after ingestion of a meal. A critical point in interpretation of the role of this reflex is that an ingested meal rapidly spreads over the whole organ or over a significant length of it. The colon contains fecal material most of the time along its entire length. Therefore, each quintessentially small location in the colon containing fecal material stimulates oral release of excitatory neurotransmitter ACh and anal release of inhibitory neurotransmitters NO/VIP, as illustrated in Figure 26. A segment distal for one focal point of mucosal stimulation is concurrently a proximal segment for stimulation from a focal point anal to it. Taken together, the circular muscle cells at all locations concurrently receive both excitatory and inhibitory neurotransmitters (Figure 26). Whether circular smooth muscle cells in a given segment contract or not depends on the relative intensity of the excitatory and inhibitory neurotransmitters released in that segment. The amplitudes of contractions at a given location will vary by the different degrees of mucosal stimulation at proximal and distal locations by the fecal material. Therefore, concurrent ascending excitation and descending inhibition is not the law of the intestines. Rather, it is a means to release concurrently the excitatory and inhibitory neurotransmitters in a short segment to produce contractions of varying amplitudes, to cause mixing/turning over and propulsion.

Take-home Messages

1. Mucosal stimulation at a focal point releases excitatory neurotransmitters orally and inhibitory neurotransmitters anally. However, this act alone does not propel anything. Postprandial propulsion occurs only when contractions occlude the lumen and propagate in the anal direction. The slow waves do not phase lock in the colon [29, 30, 189]. The RPCs regulated by these contractions largely stir and turn over the fecal material.

2. The RPCs do not compress the gut wall with sufficient amplitude to initiate descending inhibition. Descending inhibition occurs primarily in response to strong compression of the gut wall by GMCs.

3. The role of ascending excitation and descending inhibition is simply to concurrently release excitatory and inhibitory transmitters of varying amplitudes throughout the gut to generate varying amplitudes of contractions, which produce varying distances of propagations of RPCs to produce net slow distal propulsion and mixing/turning over of digesta.

4. A large part of our understanding of neuronal reflexes and circuits has come from studies on the guinea pig. While the enteric neurons in this model are easy to work with, the interpretation of the findings in this species for gut motor function in other species, specifi-

cally humans, is challenging. The guinea pig does not generate omnipresent intestinal slow waves, like other species [190–192].

5. The propulsion of an artificial pellet in an ex vivo colon segment of mice and guinea pig is often cited as evidence of propulsion by ascending excitation and descending inhibition [182, 193]. However, such propulsion does not occur in ex vivo segments of higher species, including dogs and humans. This propulsion may occur in mice and guinea pigs because they are unique in generating GMCs in ex vivo segments [13, 16].

6. The EJPs and IJPs generated in smooth muscle cells are useful indicators of the release of excitatory and inhibitory neurotransmitters to their membrane receptors. These tools work well in guinea pigs because they do not generate spontaneous slow waves. However, in an intact human gut, excitation does not occur due to an EJP, and inhibition does not occur due to an IJP. The smooth muscle cells contract because of spikes generated by excitation-contraction coupling, and they relax by the inhibition of these spikes due to excitation-inhibition coupling.

·   ·   ·   ·

Colonic Motility in Health

METHODS OF RECORDING HUMAN COLONIC MOTOR ACTIVITY AND ANALYSIS OF DATA

Silastic tubes containing side holes or solid-state transducers are widely used methods of recording human colonic motor activity. In spite of some limitations [28, 194], these methods have yielded highly useful information that is the basis of our current understanding of human colonic motor activity in health and in motility disorders. Most investigators position these tubes in the colon via the anus after colon cleansing, which alters colonic motility to some degree [38, 149, 195, 196]. However, similar effects of cleansing in controls and in patients minimize the errors in interpreting differences in findings. These methods do not record contractions that fail to occlude the lumen up to the diameter of the recording tube. However, for the colon, the non-luminal-occluding contractions have a relatively minor impact on propulsion. This limitation does not apply to GMCs, which by definition always occlude the lumen.

Colonic motor patterns are one of the most variable and unpredictable phenomena in organisms. The frequency, amplitude, and timing of all three types of contractions are variable at any given location in the colon. Overall, motor activity shows diurnal variation. Gender affects the intensity and pattern of colonic contractions. Psychological stress and physical exercise alter the motor activity and function. Together, the limitations of recording methods, heterogeneous groups of normal subjects, and unpredictable variability account for the often-conflicting findings in clinical studies. An ideal study design will include a single gender with an age difference between individuals of no more than 10 years and a solid-state transducer recording from the entire length of the colon for a minimum of 24 hours.

A computer program is needed to quantitate colonic motor activity as area under contractions (AUC). However, this number does not indicate propagation of contractions essential for propulsion. Transit time might be faster if the overall increase in colonic motor activity includes a higher frequency of propagating contractions or the mean distance of contractions increases. On the other hand, transit time may be slower if an increase in AUC is accompanied by an impairment in propagation of contractions. However, an increase in AUC might indicate a higher level of mixing/turning over of the fecal material.

Most studies define propagation as sequential occurrence of contractions over at least three adjacent recording locations, the minimum requirement. However, the distances between the recording sites vary among studies. The requirement that a contraction must propagate over at least 20 cm (about 20% of the length of the colon) will better distinguish mass movements by GMCs from slower propulsion by short-duration and long-duration RPCs. The currently used criteria (that any contraction that appears at three sequential recording sites, traveling within a wide velocity range of 0.2 to 12 cm/sec [38, 195] or any velocity greater than 0.5 cm/sec [28], is a propagating contraction) are too lenient. Using this wide range of velocity overestimates the antegrade or retrograde propagation of both types of RPCs. RPCs occur randomly at adjacent locations in the colon; the wide velocity range will include the chance occurrence of randomly occurring contractions as propagated contractions. This criterion might also give a false sense of retrograde propagation. The concept of retrograde propulsion arose from radiological observations of back and forth movements of contrast material, which is caused by bidirectional displacement of luminal contents by a strong contraction at a given location.

Take-home Message

Colonic motor activity is highly variable. Clinical study designs have come a long way from early studies, which reported data from a short distal segment of the colon recorded for one or two hours. Tighter study designs, including better stratification of patient groups, would further improve consistency between studies. No doubt, stricter designs of clinical studies are not always feasible.

CORRELATION BETWEEN COLONIC CONTRACTIONS AND PROPULSION

GMCs are the best-defined contractions in the human colon due to the lack of any ambiguity in recording them. The average frequency of GMCs in the human colon is about 6 to 10 per 24 hours, mean amplitude about 115 mmHg, mean duration about 20 seconds, and they propagate distally at a speed of about 1 cm/sec [28, 195, 197]. The definition of colonic GMCs must include amplitude of at least 100 mmHg. The calculated length of segment contracted concurrently by a GMC is about 20 cm (duration of contraction x speed of propagation). Most GMCs originate in the proximal colon and propagate a mean distance of about 45 cm [195]. Most GMCs, therefore, produce mass movements from the ascending colon to the transverse or descending colon. Only those GMCs that originate in the sigmoid colon or proximal to it and propagate up to the rectum produce the urge to defecate or act of defecation.

About two thirds of the propagating RPCs in the colon do not propel luminal contents, and one-third of the rest propel only partially [38]. The ability of a propagating RPC to propel fecal material increases with its amplitude. Therefore, most RPCs likely do not occlude the lumen of the colon, or they do not occur at uniform amplitude around the circumference to generate a uniform ringlike lumen-occluding contraction. Given that the amplitudes of RPCs are highly variable, the amplitude of a propagating RPC is highly likely to drop below a critical threshold before it reaches its maximum distance of propagation, reducing the distance and effectiveness of propulsion (see Figure 20). These factors make propulsion by RPCs highly ineffective. The lack of a strong correlation between propagating RPCs and propulsion show that colonic RPCs predominantly cause mixing and turning over of luminal contents and produce markedly slow propulsion. The long-duration contractions propagate better than the short-duration contractions and likely produce slow net propulsion over short distances [38].

The measurements of area under contractions show that the sum of all contractile activity increases steadily from the cecum to the sigmoid colon [38]. By contrast, the frequency of propagating RPCs and their mean distance of propagation decrease from the cecum to the sigmoid colon. The relatively intense RPC activity in the ascending and transverse colons results in intensive mixing/turning over of the newly arrived liquid digesta from the ileum [198, 199]. Inefficient propulsion by RPCs allows longer contact time of the newly arrived digesta to absorb water and electrolytes in these segments of the colon. As the fecal material moves to the sigmoid colon, the need for frequent turnover decreases, and so does the activity of RPCs. In fact, the RPCs would be less effective in mixing/turning over the semisolid to solid feces in the sigmoid colon anyway. These patterns of RPCs explain the slower transit in the ascending and transverse colons [199].

Take-home Messages

1. Colonic propulsion occurs primarily by GMCs.
2. RPCs in the colon are highly disorganized spatially and variable in amplitude from one contraction to the next, requiring computer-based analysis to quantitate the area under contractions and mean propagation distances.
3. The RPCs primarily turn over fecal material for uniform exposure to the absorptive mucosal surface. Total RPC activity decreases from the ascending to the sigmoid colon.

DIURNAL VARIATIONS OF HUMAN COLONIC MOTOR ACTIVITY

The overall colonic motor activity, (area under contractions; AUC) as well as the frequency of GMCs, exhibit diurnal variation [28, 34, 154, 197, 200–202] (Figure 27). The overall activity reduces by about half throughout the colon in females and males during sleep. The reduction is less in the rectosigmoid colon of male subjects [28]. The frequency of GMCs reduces by about 80% during

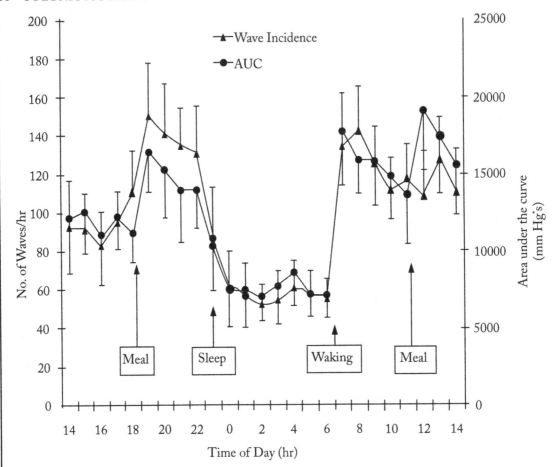

FIGURE 27: Twenty-four-hour profile of the area under contractions (AUC) and the total number of contractions in healthy humans. Both parameters increased after ingestion of a 1000-kCal meal at 6:00 PM, on waking up in the morning, and after 400-kCal breakfast. Waves means contractions. (Reproduced with permission from Rao et al., *Am J Physiol Gastrointest Liver Physiol*, 280: G629–G639, 2001 [28].)

sleep [203]—the nocturnal GMCs occur primarily in the ascending colon [200]. The reduction in the frequency of propagated RPCs relates to the depth of sleep [200]. However, the propagating RPCs or even GMCs in the ascending colon appear transiently during nocturnal arousal from deep sleep and during the REM stage of sleep.

An obvious reason for depression of colonic motor activity during sleep is to slow down fecal transit, which prevents awakening at night for bowel movement. The motor activity of the upper gut also decreases during sleep [204]. Respiratory and cardiovascular functions are similarly correlated with sleep stages [205–207].

Colonic motor activity, including the frequency of GMCs, significantly increases upon awakening in the morning, which sometimes induces the urge to defecate followed by defecation [28, 34, 197]. The stimulus for increase of motor activity during nocturnal arousals, the REM stage of sleep, and awakening in the morning comes from the CNS via the autonomic neurons, but we do not know the precise mechanisms. It is likely that central activity stimulates the parasympathetic neurons to activate the enteric cholinergic excitatory neurons. The enteric neurons may have accumulated ChAT or ACh in vesicles during low activity in sleep to mount a robust contractile response during nocturnal arousal, REM, or awakening in the morning.

Take-home Messages

1. Colonic motor activity, including RPCs and GMCs, exhibits diurnal variation to slow down transit during sleep.
2. Colonic motor activity increases sharply on awakening, which may result in the urge to defecate.

GASTROCOLONIC REFLEX/RESPONSE

The increase in colonic motor activity following a meal—especially in the morning when the sigmoid colon and rectum are likely full—is a primitive reflex to prod the colon to empty in preparation for the entry of new digesta [22, 43, 44, 208–211]. Most clinical and animal studies show that this response occurs in the whole colon and lasts less than 2 hours [212, 213]. A pronounced increase in sigmoid motor activity—particularly when it includes GMCs—induces an urge to defecate. Infants and newborns display this reflex prominently. Adults may adapt to ignore it.

Studies on experimental animals suggest that the vago-vagal reflex mediates the gastrocolonic response to ingestion of a meal [214, 215]. Electrical stimulation of efferent thoracic vagal fibers stimulates colonic motor activity [216]. The efferent vagal neurons synapse on enteric neurons to enhance the release of ACh, which in turn stimulates excitation-contraction coupling in circular smooth muscle cells to contract them. Clinical studies show that cholinergic receptor antagonists, interference with calcium mobilization by octylonium bromide, or calcium channel blockers (nifedipine and verapamil) block the gastrocolonic response to eating a meal [42, 43, 217, 218], which confirms the roles of cholinergic excitatory motor neurons and excitation-contraction coupling in gastrocolonic response.

The ingestion of a regular meal containing fat releases cholecystokinin (CCK) from endocrine cells in the duodenum and jejunum. However, systemic administration of CCK-8 [22] or cerulean—an analog of CCK-8—to attain its plasma levels within the range achieved by ingestion of a 1000 kCal meal has no significant effect on colonic motor activity in any part of the human colon [208]. In addition, the inhibition of CCK-1 receptors by loxiglumide [208] or dexloxiglumide [219] does not block the gastrocolonic response to ingestion of a meal or transient increase in colonic propulsion, respectively. Therefore, the postprandial physiologic concentrations of CCK in healthy subjects do not affect colonic motor activity or function. However, pharmacologic doses of CCK-8 stimulate colonic motor activity [208]. The safe administration of CCK-8 in humans makes it a useful tool to investigate the potential loci of defect in regulatory mechanisms in motility disorders. CCK acts on presynaptic neurons to release ACh [22], which stimulates contractions. A defect in the motor response to CCK suggests a possible impairment in ACh synthesis/release and/or a defect in excitation-contraction coupling in smooth muscle cells (see Figures 10 and 11).

The evaluation of gastrocolonic response is an effective tool to investigate abnormalities in the release of ACh and excitation-contraction coupling in colonic motility disorders. However, this test cannot pinpoint whether the abnormal response is due to a defect in the synthesis/release of ACh or in the cell-signaling pathways of excitation-contraction coupling. The increase of contractile activity in the sigmoid colon by the short-acting cholinesterase inhibitor edrophonium chloride is greater than in the rest of the colon, suggesting that it might contain a greater number of ChAT-containing neurons or that these neurons may express higher levels of ChAT [220].

Take-home Messages

1. The ingestion of a meal (~1000 kCal) enhances colonic motor activity for about two hours.
2. Vago-vagal reflex mediates the gastrocolonic response. Efferent vagal nerves stimulate the enteric cholinergic neurons to enhance the release of ACh, resulting in an increase of colonic motor activity.
3. The physiological increase of plasma CCK does not contribute to the gastrocolonic response. However, pharmacological doses of CCK increase colonic contractions by releasing ACh from the enteric motor neurons.

DEFECATION

Perfect defecation means painless and complete evacuation of the rectum and part of the sigmoid and descending colons in a short period after receiving a few minutes of warning. Under resting conditions, tonic contraction of the internal anal sphincter (regulated by myogenic mechanisms) and tonic contractions of the external anal sphincter and puborectalis muscle (regulated by central mechanisms) maintain continence. Defecation is a three-step process. (1) Issue a warning of impending defecation to allow subjects to find a safe and convenient place. (2) Relax the anal sphincters and puborectalis muscle for resistance-free passage of stool. (3) Induce a mass movement to accomplish defecation in a reasonably short period. The following considerations explain the defecation process.

1. RPCs play little role in evacuation during defecation. Propulsion by this type of contraction is very sluggish in the colon. The distal colon would require several hours to empty solely by RPCs; this is not acceptable. In addition, RPCs do not produce descending inhibition to relax the internal anal sphincter. However, RPCs may gradually fill up the rectum. The rectum accommodates slow filling without sending sensory signals to the higher centers. In this case, the urge to defecate may occur after a long delay when rectal filling exceeds its accommodative capacity.

2. GMCs play a critical role in normal defecation: they rapidly propel luminal contents over long distances to provide the force for expulsion of feces within a short period. Usually, a

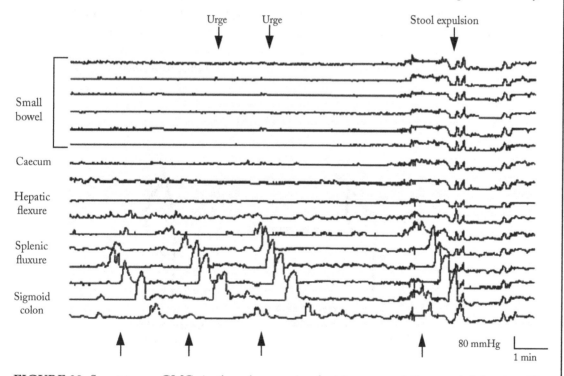

FIGURE 28: Spontaneous GMCs in the colon associated with urges to defecate and defecation. The first three GMCs (shown by upward arrows) started near the splenic flexure and terminated in the sigmoid colon. The second and third GMCs caused urges to defecate. The fourth GMC propagated to the end of the colon and caused defecation. The simultaneous increase of pressure at all recording locations during defecation indicates straining. (Reproduced with permission from Bampton et al., *Am J Gastroenterol*, 95: 1027–1035, 2000 [36].)

group of GMCs begins in the ascending or the descending colon, but they stop short of the rectum (Figure 28) [36]. These predefecation GMCs bring the fecal material to the descending/sigmoid colon and rapidly fill up the rectum. The internal and external anal sphincters remain closed (Figure 29). The filling of the rectum, with the internal and external anal sphincters closed, distends the rectum, which sends the signal for urge to defecate to the CNS via the visceral sensory nerves [8, 36]. Rapid distension of a balloon in the rectum mimics this urge to defecate [221]. There is generally a window of up to about 15 minutes to evacuate after the initial warning.

3. The assumption of squatting or sitting position straightens the anorectal angle to allow easy passage of the feces (Figure 29).

4. The sensory mechanisms in the upper anal canal sense the fecal contents as gas, liquid, or solid [222].

5. During the final phase of defecation, a GMC or GMCs propagate up to the rectum, pushing feces into the anal canal. These GMCs produce descending inhibition of the internal anal sphincter via the enteric interneurons and inhibitory motor neurons (see section on

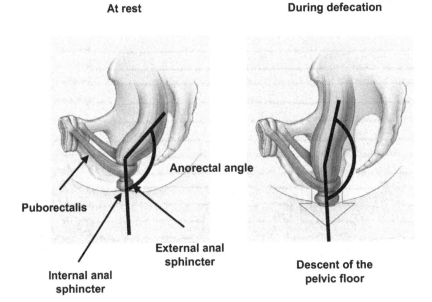

FIGURE 29: Pelvic floor function during defecation. (A) At rest, the closure of internal and external sphincters as well as the acute anal-rectal angle maintains continence. (B) The squatting position and voluntary relaxation of the puborectalis muscle and external sphincter allow the passage of feces pushed by a GMC. (Reproduced with modification from Lembo, A, and Camilleri, M, *N Engl J Med*, 349(14): 1360–1368, 2003 [497].)

descending inhibition), which relaxes the internal anal sphincter [223]. The puborecta-lis muscle and external anal sphincters relax under voluntary control (Figure 29), further straightening the anorectal angle with perineal descent to allow expulsion of feces. This sequence may repeat a few times for complete evacuation as far up as the middle colon. The pressure in the external anal sphincter returns to baseline to resume continence.

Valsalva maneuver (straining) during the final phase of defecation increases intra-abdominal pressure to squeeze the rectum and aid in the expulsion of feces, much like squeezing toothpaste. However, in the absence of GMCs, the Valsalva maneuver by itself causes imperfect defecation. First, it empties primarily the stools in the rectum, causing small volume of fecal expulsion. Second, compression of the rectum by increase in abdominal pressure does not induce descending inhibition; only distension or a strong contraction, such as a GMC, produces descending inhibition.

Take-home Messages

1. GMCs in the sigmoid colon fill up the rectum while the anal sphincters are closed, causing an urge to defecate.
2. Subsequent GMCs that propagate up to the rectum produce descending inhibition, which relaxes the internal anal sphincter.
3. The puborectalis muscle and external anal sphincter relax under voluntary control while GMC expels the feces.
4. Fecal expulsion by Valsalva maneuver requires straining to push feces through the anal sphincters due to the lack of adequate descending inhibition.

WHAT CAUSES THE RANDOM GENERATION OF GMCs?

While we do not know the complete answer, a number of observations and pharmacological experi-ments provide significant clues to the generation of GMCs.

1. Voluntary actions do not generate GMCs. However, the incidence of GMCs decreases during sleep, and GMCs do not occur under anesthesia. By contrast, the probability of occurrence of GMC increases after a meal or on awakening in the morning. Finally, intra-cerebroventricular (ICV) administration of thyrotrpophin releasing hormone by a cannula in the left ventricle stimulates a colonic GMC (Figure 30A). Taken together, the activa-tion of neurons in the lower brain stimulates colonic GMCs, but this action is not under voluntary control.

A.

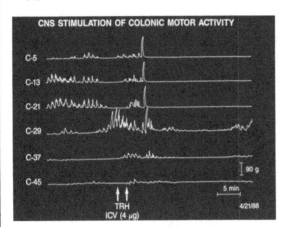

B.

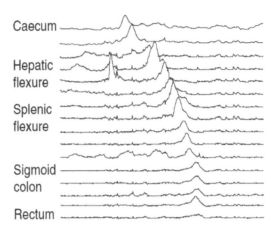

FIGURE 30: Central stimulation of GMCs. (A) An intracerebroventricular administration of thyrotrophin-releasing hormone stimulated a GMC in the dog colon. (B) Electrical stimulation of the S3 sacral nerve increased the daily frequency of GMCs in a patient with slow-transit defecation. One of these GMCs is shown in this figure. This GMC started in the ascending colon, but its amplitude decreased in the sigmoid colon. (Reproduced with permission from Dinning et al. and Cook, IJ, *Colorectal Disease*, 9: 123–132, 2007 [224].)

2. S2 and S3 sacral nerve stimulation increases the frequency of GMCs twofold throughout the colon (Figure 30B) [224]. The central stimulation of GMC likely works through the parasympathetic outflow.

3. The stimulation of mucosal nerve endings by bisacodyl, a mucosal irritant contact laxative, stimulates colonic GMCs [225–227]. We do not know whether bisacodyl stimulates intrinsic sensory neurons or the extrinsic sensory neurons (vago-vagal reflex) to stimulate GMCs. Regardless, each pathway as well as sacral nerve stimulation and central stimulation by thyrotrophin-releasing hormone converge on the enteric motor neurons to release ACh. Supramaximal accumulation of ACh at the neuromuscular junction activates excitation-contraction coupling in circular muscle cells to stimulate GMCs (see earlier section on GMCs). Neostigmine and edrophonium chloride stimulate GMCs also by accumulation of ACh at the neuromuscular junction [8, 134, 220] (Figure 31).

4. Fermentation by anaerobic bacteria breaks down undigested carbohydrates into short-chain fatty acids. The infusion of short-chain fatty acids into the human ileum results in abdominal cramping and an urge to defecate [228]. The investigators did not record colonic motility in this study, but these symptoms are typical of colonic GMCs. However, they found that ileal infusion of volatile fatty acids in dogs stimulates GMCs that propagate right up

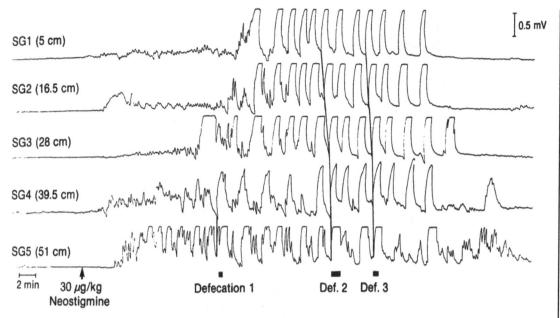

SG1 (5 cm)

SG2 (16.5 cm)

SG3 (28 cm)

SG4 (39.5 cm)

SG5 (51 cm)

0.5 mV

2 min   30 µg/kg   Defecation 1   Def. 2   Def. 3
          Neostigmine

FIGURE 31: Stimulation of GMCs in canine colon by intravenous administration of 30 µg/kg neostigmine, a cholinesterase inhibitor. Neostigmine stimulated a series of GMCs, three of which (connected by solid lines) resulted in defecations. SG = strain gauge transducer. The number in parenthesis indicates the distance of the transducer from the cecum. (Reproduced with permission from Karaus, M, and Sarna, SK, *Gastroenterology*, 92: 925–933, 1987 [8].)

to the terminal ileum and presumably into the colon to generate the urge to defecate [229] (Figure 32A). Animal studies in rats show that colonic infusion of short-chain fatty acids indeed stimulates GMCs in the proximal colon that propagate all the way to the distal colon [230] (Figure 32B). Short-chain fatty acids in the colon stimulate the release of 5-HT from the enterochromafin cells. 5-HT acts on 5-HT$_3$ receptors on vagal afferents neurons to stimulate vago-vagal reflex. The efferent vagal nerves synapse on nicotinic receptors on enteric motor neurons to release ACh, which stimulates GMCs [230].

5. The stimulation of GMCs by short-chain fatty acids can be blocked by 1) mucosal application of lidocane, which desensitizes nerve endings, 2) intraluminal application of 5-HT$_3$ receptor antagonist, 3) bilateral vagotomy, or 4) intravenous administration of hexamethonium or atropine. These findings suggest that short-chain fatty acids use the vago-vagal reflex, rather than the intrinsic neuronal reflex involving ISNs and interneurons, to stimulate GMCs.

6. Perfusion of long-chain oleic acid—a common dietary constituent—in the ascending colon

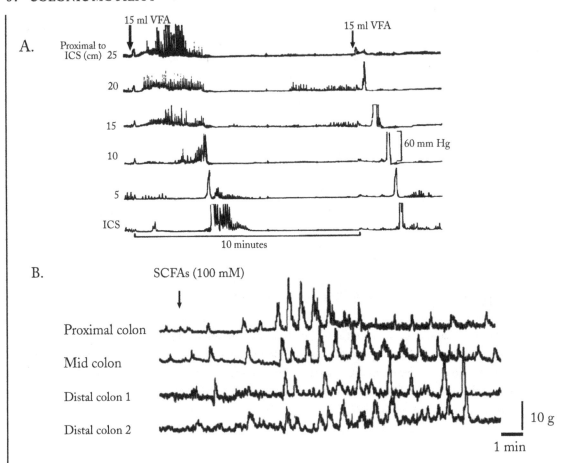

FIGURE 32: Intraluminal administration of volatile fatty acids (VFA) stimulates GMCs. (A) Intraluminal administration of short-chain fatty acids in an isolated loop of ileum and colon with intact extrinsic innervations stimulated a GMC that propagated to the ileocolonic sphincter (ICS). (Reproduced with permission from Kamath et al. and Phillips, SF, *Am J Physiol Gastrointesti Liver Physiol*, 16: g427–g433, 1987 [229].) (B) Intraluminal administration of 100 mM short-chain fatty acids stimulated a group of GMCs in the proximal colon that propagated to the distal colon. (Reproduced with permission from Fukumoto et al. and Takahashi, T, *Am J Physiol Regul Integr Comp Physiol*, 284: R1269–R1276, 2003 [230].)

stimulates GMCs that start near the cecum and propagate in the anal direction (Figure 33). The GMCs accelerate colonic transit, associate with abdominal cramping, and induce defecation [231]. This model mimics steatorrhea. Control infusions of saline have no effect.

7.   Strenuous physical exercise after a meal stimulates GMCs [232]. The ingestion of a meal increases colonic motor activity. Most of the postprandial increase in motor activity is of nonpropagating RPCs because the patients lie in bed during this test for manometric re-

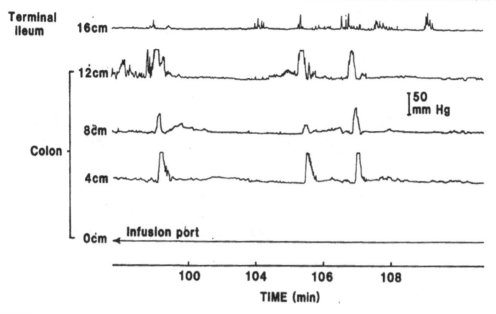

FIGURE 33: Perfusion of oleic acid into the ascending colon stimulates GMCs that start near the cecum and propagate in the anal direction. (Reproduced with permission from Spiller et al. and Phillips,
SF, *Gastroenterology*, 91: 100–107, 1986 [231].)

cording. However, if patients are mobile after a meal, the frequency of GMC increases, producing mass movements [233]. Taken together, somatic activity in the postprandial state
promotes the stimulation of colonic GMCs (mass movements).

8. Excessive absorbable or nonabsorbable fluids in the colon—including those secreted from
    the small intestine by oral laxatives—stimulate GMCs [149, 234, 235].

Take-home Messages

1. Vagovagal reflex may play a prominent role in the generation of colonic GMCs.
2. Short-chain fatty acids generated by bacterial fermentation of carbohydrates in the ascend-
    ing colon may be a major dietary source of stimulation of GMCs in the colon. This works
    well because fermentation produces short-chain fatty acids with delay, which allows time
    for absorption of water and electrolytes in the ascending colon before a GMC propels them
    by mass movement.
3. Malabsorption of fats is also a dietary source of stimulation of colonic GMCs.
4. The release of 5-HT in the colon utilizes vago-vagal reflex, rather than the enteric reflexes,
    to stimulate GMCs.

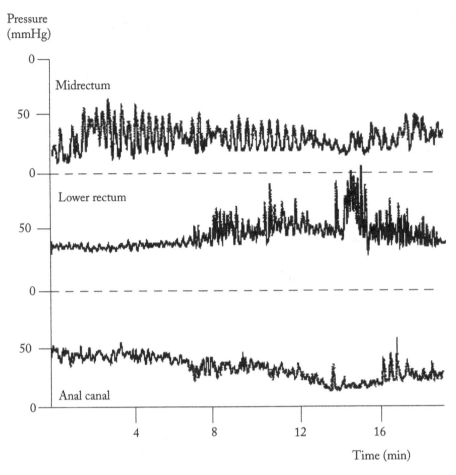

FIGURE 34: Rectal motor complexes in the mid and lower rectums. (Reproduced with permission from Ronholt et al. and Chritiansen, J, *Dis Colon Rectum*, 42:1551–1558, 1999 [237].)

5.   Several physiological stimuli, such as somatic activity, stimulate GMCs when ingestion of a meal has primed the vago-vagal reflex.

ANORECTAL MOTOR ACTIVITY

Anorectal motor activity plays a critical role in maintaining continence. Findings from several studies using the manometric method of recording show marked variations in details, such as amplitudes, durations, and frequencies of contractions as well as in the effects of meal ingestion and sleep on these parameters [236–244]. The following points represent consensus related to anorectal motor function.

1. The resting anal pressure (about 70 mmHg) is greater than the resting rectal pressure (about 30 to 40 mmHg). This gradient is helpful in maintaining continence.
2. The rectum generates periodic bursts of contractions: rectal motor complex (RMC) (Figure 34). Each burst of contractions lasts about 5 to 10 minutes during the awake state and recurs at a frequency of about 0.5/hour. RMCs may occur more frequently in the distal rectum than in the mid or proximal rectum. The contractions occur at a frequency of about 2 to 3 cycles per minute.
3. Most parameters of RMCs decrease during sleep and increase after a meal. We do not understand the roles of RMCs in maintaining continence.
4. The anal canal shows transient spontaneous relaxations that relate loosely to contractions in the rectum.

Colonic Motility Dysfunction

The colon is the last major organ in the gastrointestinal tract. Therefore, it plays a critical role in regulating the frequency of defecation and consistency of stools. The two primary symptoms of colonic motility dysfunction are altered bowel habits (constipation, diarrhea) and intermittent abdominal cramping. Additional symptoms include straining, urgency, feeling of incomplete evacuation, passage of mucus, bloating or feeling of abdominal distension, and postprandial exacerbation of symptoms. The following sections discuss the symptoms of specific motility disorders affecting the colon, the motor correlates of these symptoms, and the cellular and molecular mechanisms of dysfunction, following a brief discussion of how physiological or pathologic motor activity produces the sensation of abdominal pain.

GMCs AND VISCERAL PAIN OF GUT ORIGIN

The link between abnormal motility and altered bowel habits is obvious. However, it is not always apparent how a motor event in the gut can be the source of abdominal cramping. The sensation of pain requires three components (Figure 35):

1. A noxious mechanical or chemical stimulus to generate an afferent signal
2. Afferent sensory neurons to transmit the signal to the CNS, and
3. The CNS circuitry, which processes this signal and sends the information to the higher centers for perception of pain.

There are two types of mechanical events in the gut: compression of the gut wall by contractions and distension of the receiving segment during mass movements. Earlier sections showed that the amplitude and duration of a GMC are twofold to threefold greater than those of RPCs. The longer duration of a GMC means that it concurrently contracts a long-segment of the gut (about 20 cm in the colon). In addition, a GMC propagates rapidly over long distances and propels a large bolus ahead of it, which distends the receiving segment (Figure 36). By contrast, an RPC contracts a short segment (about 1 to 2 cm). RPCs move luminal contents back and forth with slow net distal propulsion and do not cause distension of the receiving segment (Figure 36).

Nociceptive Signaling Pathways

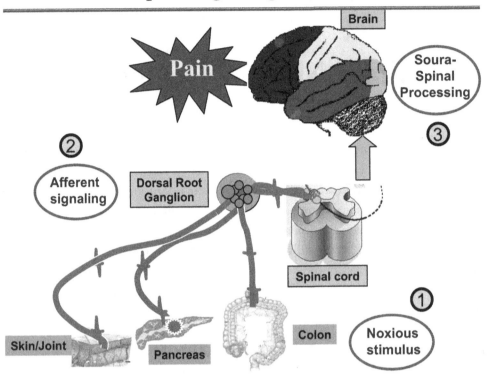

FIGURE 35: Cartoon showing three essential components for perception of pain. (1) A noxious signal from a peripheral organ. (2) Afferent neurons to transmit this signal to the CNS. (3) Processing of this signal in the CNS and sending it to the higher centers for perception.

The primary afferent fibers with mechanosensitive nerve endings in the muscularis externa respond to circumferential stretch and send the signal to the CNS via the afferent 1st- and 2nd-order splanchnic neurons [245–247]. The afferent signal is proportional to the degree of distension [23]. These mechanoreceptors respond similarly to compression of the gut wall by a GMC and its distension by an intraluminal balloon, and the two signals are additive.

Taken together, this means that a GMC will generate a much-higher-intensity afferent signal than an RPC due to its stronger compression of the gut wall and larger mechanosensitive field. A recent study showed that the occurrence of a GMC in the small intestine generates a pseudoaffective signal, but small intestinal RPCs do not [23].

GMCs occur spontaneously several times a day in healthy subjects and do not produce the sensation of pain. The reason for lack of painful sensation is that the afferent signal generated by a

ETIOLOGY OF ABDOMINAL PAIN OF MOTILITY ORIGIN

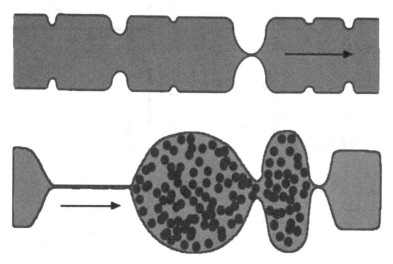

FIGURE 36: Differential effects of RPCs and GMCs on the compression of the gut wall, propulsion of luminal contents, and distension of the descending segments. (Top diagram) The RPCs do not strongly compress the colon wall and they do not produce mass movements to distend the receiving segment. (Bottom diagram) A GMC strongly compresses a long segment of the colon. Its rapid distal propagation produces mass movement, which distends the receiving segment.

GMC in health is below the nociceptive threshold (Figure 37A). However, this signal may exceed the nociceptive threshold and be perceived as painful under the following scenarios.

1. The amplitudes of GMCs increase due to neuromuscular dysfunction so that the afferent signal generated by them exceeds the nociceptive threshold (Figure 37B). This scenario is similar to that in which balloon distension in the rectum or sigmoid colon exceeds the nociceptive threshold.

2. The development of hypersensitivity in afferent neurons or impairment of CNS processing effectively lowers the nociceptive threshold (Figure 37C) so that GMCs of normal amplitude exceed it and induce painful sensation.

3. Due to impairment of descending inhibition, the descending segment generates tone and sends afferent signals to the CNS. The combined afferent signals, due to strong compression by GMC and distension of the receiving segment, exceed the nociceptive threshold to induce the sensation of pain in the CNS (Figure 37D). This scenario develops particularly when the sphincters, such as the anal sphincters, fail to relax. In this case, a GMC attempts to push feces against a closed sphincter, but due to the closure, the intervening segment

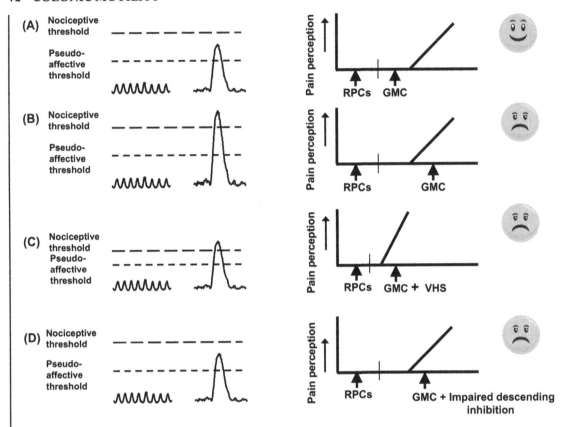

FIGURE 37: Cartoon shows the conditions under which GMCs generate afferent signals that exceed the nociceptive threshold. The x-axis in diagrams on the right side indicates the intensity of afferent signal. (A) In normal state, the afferent signal generated by a GMC is above the pseudoaffective threshold but below the nociceptive threshold. The descending inhibition prevents the receiving segment from generating tone and hence afferent signals. No sensation of pain develops. (B) Due to enteric neuromuscular dysfunction, the amplitude of GMCs increases so that the afferent signals generated by them exceed the nociceptive threshold, and painful sensation results. (C) Visceral hypersensitivity of the afferent neurons or impaired processing of signals in the CNS effectively lowers the nociceptive threshold so that the afferent signal generated by a GMC of normal amplitude exceeds the threshold for perception of pain. (D) Due to impairment of descending inhibition, the receiving segment generates tone and sends afferent signals. These signals add to those generated by the GMC. The combined signal exceeds the nociceptive threshold to induce the sensation of pain.

balloons up. Note that, in normal subjects, the release of NO by descending inhibition prevents the generation of tone in the receiving segment, preventing it from generating the afferent signals [23].

Take-home Messages

1. GMCs are the essential peripheral stimuli that generate the sensation of pain of gut origin.
2. Each GMC from its beginning to its termination lasts for a short period of a few minutes. This explains the sensation of short-lived intermittent abdominal cramping.
3. GMCs can start anywhere in the colon and propagate to various distances. This suggests that the pain may localize in any quadrant of the abdomen or migrate among different quadrants.
4. Abdominal cramping may occur in the absence of visceral hypersensitivity or impaired CNS processing due to enhancement of GMC amplitudes or impairment of descending inhibition.
5. Visceral hypersensitivity by itself does not cause pain. There has to be a stimulus, such as a GMC, that generates an afferent signal for perception of pain.

IRRITABLE BOWEL SYNDROME

The prevalence of IBS is about 11% to 14% in the general population in North America [248–250]. About 70% of IBS patients consulting physicians in Western countries are females [251]. Rome II criteria define IBS as having abdominal pain/discomfort along with at least two of the following three features. (1) Defecation relieves pain/discomfort. (2) Onset of pain associates with an abnormal frequency of stools (more than three times per day or fewer than three times per week). (3) Onset of pain associates with a change in the form of the stool [252]. Additional supportive symptoms in IBS patients include straining, urgency, feeling of incomplete evacuation, passage of mucus, bloating, feeling of abdominal distension, and postprandial exacerbation of symptoms. Altered colonic motor function may result in constipation (constipation-predominant IBS [IBS-C]), diarrhea (diarrhea predominant IBS [IBS-D]), or alternating constipation and diarrhea IBS (IBS-C/D). In addition, recent studies show that about 10% to 25% of patients develop the symptoms of IBS after an episode of severe or prolonged enteric inflammation (postinfectious IBS [IBS-PI]).

Diarrhea-Predominant IBS

In addition to intermittent abdominal cramping, IBS-D patients have one or more of the following symptoms: (1) more than three bowel movements per day, (2) loose (mushy) or watery stools, and (3) urgency of defecation.

Colonic Motor Dysfunction in IBS-D Patients

IBS-D patients presenting with abdominal pain and diarrhea show a several-fold increase in the frequency and amplitude of spontaneous GMCs, compared with healthy controls [22]. Several of the GMCs in IBS-D patients result in defecation during manometric recordings, indicating urgency. The transit time of radiopaque pellets from the cecum to defecation in these patients was several-fold faster than in controls [22]. About 90% of the GMCs in patients were associated with the sensation of intermittent short-lived abdominal cramping. Diarrhea usually occurred after breakfast, and cramping subsided after defecation. The GMCs in the healthy cohort did not produce the

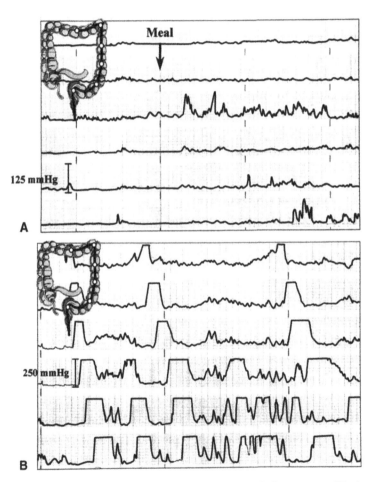

FIGURE 38: The ingestion of a meal stimulates GMCs in IBS-D patients (B), but not in healthy control subjects (A). The amplitude of GMCs in IBS-D patients is more than twice that of healthy controls.

sensation of abdominal cramping. The intensity of RPCs (measured as area under contractions) in IBS-D patients was not different from that in healthy controls, except in the descending colon, where it was greater.

The above findings demonstrate a primary role of motility dysfunction—an increase in the frequency and amplitude of GMCs-in generating the symptoms of diarrhea, urgency and abdominal cramping in IBS-D patients. These findings also show that RPCs may have little role in the induction of these symptoms. As indicated earlier, RPCs are essential in frequent and regular turning over of fecal material, thus allowing uniform and extensive exposure of the fecal material to the mucosa for absorption of water and electrolytes. However, rapid propulsion by increase in the frequency of GMCs deprives the fecal material of adequate exposure to mucosa, resulting in loose stools. IBS-D patients do not have impaired absorptive function.

The above group of patients experienced daily symptoms of abdominal bloating, cramping, urgency, and frequent bowel movements ranging from 4 to more than 15 per day for more than 6 months. Therefore, these patients represent cases of moderate to severe IBS-D. The classification of IBS-D patients by Rome III criteria is liberal [253]. As a result, studies that select patients by strict Rome II or Rome III criteria find an increase in the frequency of GMCs in IBS-D patients, which may not reach statistical significance [39]. The colonic transit in a wider population of IBS-D patients is faster than in controls [254–261] but not as much as in patients of the above study with severe symptoms of IBS-D [22]. However, the association between frequent GMCs and faster propulsion and sensation of abdominal cramping with most GMCs in IBS-D patients is present in almost all studies. The relief in abdominal cramping following a bowel movement is due to the lack of a stimulus in the distal colon to generate GMCs.

As shown in Figure 37B, a significant increase in the amplitude of GMCs in IBS-D patients by itself should be enough to increase compression of the colon wall to above the nociceptive threshold. However, a subset of IBS-D patients show hypersensitivity to colorectal distension by a balloon [247, 262–267], which would increase the susceptibility of inducing abdominal cramping by GMCs (see Figure 37C).

Take-home Messages

1. The frequency and amplitude of GMCs increase significantly in IBS-D patients.
2. These increases relate to the severity of symptoms of abdominal cramping and bowel movements per day.
3. The increase in the amplitude of GMCs by itself may be sufficient to induce the sensation of abdominal cramping in IBS-D patients. Concurrent visceral hypersensitivity exaggerates this sensation.

4. The relief of abdominal cramping may relate to reduction in the incidence of GMCs following defecation.

5. However, if a GMC occurs in the absence of feces in the sigmoid colon, it might initiate an urge to defecate, giving the sensation of incomplete evacuation.

Constipation-Predominant IBS, Slow-Transit Constipation, Idiopathic Constipation, and Constipation Due to Pelvic Floor Dysfunction

According to the Rome II criteria, IBS-C patients present with one or more of the following symptoms: (1) fewer than three bowel movements per week, (2) hard or lumpy stools, (3) straining during bowel movements, and (4) intermittent short-lived abdominal cramping. The patients with IBS-C differ from those with other subtypes of constipation primarily by the absence of abdominal cramping. However, this discrimination is not absolute: non-IBS-C constipated patients may also have abdominal cramps, albeit less frequently. This section discusses all subtypes of constipation together. This does not imply that constipation in different subtypes has the same etiology or that it is manageable by a common approach. The discussion of the subtypes of constipation together highlights the overlapping motor dysfunctions that lead to straining, hard stools, and fewer than three stools per week.

The severity of constipation and types of symptoms differ widely among patients within the same classification. This heterogeneity has resulted in inconsistent findings among clinical studies, which makes it difficult to formulate hypotheses for mechanistic studies.

Colonic Motor Dysfunction in IBS-C, Slow-Transit Constipation (STC), Idiopathic Constipation, and Pelvic Floor Dysfunction (PFD) Patients

The amplitude and frequency of GMCs in IBS-C, STC, idiopathic constipation, and PFD patients are less than half of those in normal subjects; in severe cases of constipation, GMCs are totally absent or scarce [203, 268–272]. The suppression of GMCs in constipation may be pancolonic or confined to the distal colon. Ambulatory 24-hour recordings from STC patients show depression of the overall contractile activity of the colon throughout the day. These patients also show suppression in normal increase of colonic motor activity after awakening in the morning [271].

The frequency and amplitude of GMCs in the colon of patients with constipation due to pelvic floor dysfunction do not differ from those in normal subjects [272]. However, the GMCs are noticeably absent or reduced in frequency when patients feel the urge to defecate (Figure 39). The urge to defecate in these patients may come from the accumulation of feces in the sigmoid colon or rectum due to RPCs. In the absence of GMCs propagating to the rectum, the descending inhibition and the propulsive force for defecation are absent in constipated patients. Hard straining may not be enough to push feces against the closed internal and external anal sphincters. Additional struc-

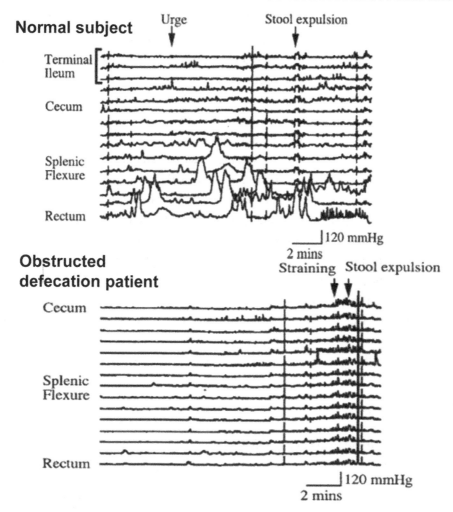

Normal subject

Urge

Stool expulsion

Terminal Ileum

Cecum

Splenic Flexure

Rectum

120 mmHg

2 mins

Obstructed defecation patient

Straining Stool expulsion

Cecum

Splenic Flexure

Rectum

120 mmHg

2 mins

FIGURE 39: GMCs are notably absent, fewer in number, or do not propagate up to the rectum prior to and at the time of defecation in patients with obstructed (pelvic floor dysfunction) defecation. In the absence of a driving force for expulsion of feces and descending inhibition, straining causes incomplete evacuation. (Reproduced with permission from Dinning et al. and Cook, IJ, *Gastroenterol*, 127: 49–56, 2004 [272].)

tural impairments in the pelvic floor function may exacerbate the difficulty in stool expulsion in some patients.

Pelvic floor dysfunction in constipation may partly be due to impaired motility function of the sigmoid colon. The internal anal sphincter relaxation depends on descending inhibitory signal generated by GMCs propagating up to it. In addition, strong compression by GMCs generates the afferent signal (urge) to relax voluntarily the puborectalis muscle and external anal sphincter. The decrease in the frequency and amplitude of GMCs in constipated patients would compromise both aspects of pelvic floor function. Additional abnormalities in enteric neuromuscular function or in autonomic nerves regulating the puborectalis and external anal sphincter may worsen constipation in these patients. We do not know whether abnormalities in GMCs and impairments in pelvic floor regulation occur independently or whether one leads to the other. Rectal motor complexes are absent in some constipated patients, indicating enteric neuromuscular dysfunction (Figure 40).

The total incidence of RPCs measured as area under contractions in constipation is variable; it depends on the severity of constipation. The area under contractions in patients with normal colonic transit, with moderately slow transit, or in patients with IBS-C is higher than that in healthy controls [273]. Note that these data, obtained by a wireless capsule, have less fidelity than those obtained by manometric tube. Another study, using the manometric method of recording, found that the area under contractions in slow-transit constipation is less than that in healthy subjects throughout the day (Figure 41). It is worth noting that, in the absence of GMCs or a reduction in their frequency, colonic propulsion occurs primarily by propagating RPCs. Therefore, having more RPCs does not necessarily mean that propulsion will be faster. Propulsion is faster only if the incidence of propagating RPCs increases. These data are not available. However, as noted earlier, the contribution of RPCs to colonic propulsion is relatively minor. They may influence the consistency of stools by regulating the intensity of turning over of luminal contents.

Take-home Messages

1. The amplitude and frequency of GMCs decrease significantly in constipated patients.
2. The severity of constipation relates to the intensity of suppression of GMCs.

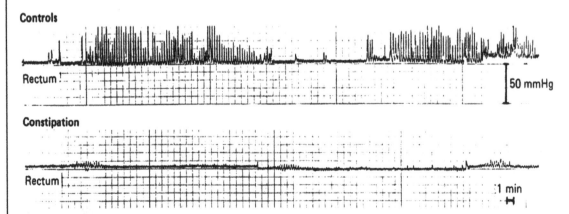

FIGURE 40: The rectal motor complexes were nearly absent in a patient with constipation. (Reproduced with permission from Waldron, DJ, *Gut*, 31: 1284–1288, 1990 [498].)

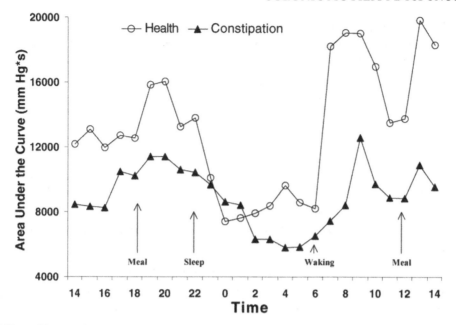

FIGURE 41: Twenty-four-hour mapping of total colonic motor activity (area under contractions) in slow-transit constipation patients. The total colonic motor activity is suppressed in constipated patients throughout the day. Note that the increases in motor activity after a meal and on awakening in the morning show impairments in patients, compared with normal subjects. (Reproduced with permission from Rao et al., *Am J Gastroenterol*, 99: 2405–2416, 2004 [271].)

3. The suppression of GMCs in the sigmoid colon will impair pelvic floor function, adding to the severity of constipation.

4. There is no consistent change in the parameters of propagating or nonpropagating RPCs in any type of constipation.

5. Diagnosis of motility disturbances in IBS-D, IBS-C, slow-transit constipation, idiopathic constipation, and obstructed defecation could be made simply by analyzing the frequency of GMCs over 24 hours, their amplitude, duration, distance of propagation, and point of origin in the whole colon. These analyses do not require a computer program. Ambulatory recordings with solid-state transducers would provide more physiological data.

6. GMCs are a reliable biomarker of both primary symptoms of IBS: altered bowel habits and abdominal cramping.

7. The Rome criteria to subdivide IBS patients into different groups are subjective and symptom based. They have not received universal acceptance after three revisions. A mechanism-based criterion, using 24-hour recordings of GMCs, might be more objective. The inclusion of objective criteria would spur mechanistic studies followed by development of therapeutic agents to normalize dysfunctional proteins.

Alternating Constipation/Diarrhea IBS

The symptoms of patients with IBS-C/D alternate randomly between those of IBS-C and IBS-D. We do not know the precise motor patterns during the two opposite conditions of motility function. However, one can extrapolate from what we know about the motor patterns in IBS-C and IBS-D patients that the frequency of GMCs fluctuates from one extreme to the other in IBS-C/D group: when the frequency is above normal, diarrhea results; when it is below normal, constipation results.

Postinfectious IBS

Clinical observations show that a subset (about 10% to 25%) of the subjects exposed to enteric infections in an individual or community setting go on to develop predominantly the symptoms of IBS-D [274–280]. Two major risk factors predispose individuals to developing postinfectious IBS symptoms following an enteric infection: (1) enteritis lasting more than 3 weeks significantly increases the risk for developing IBS-PI over a duration lasting less than 1 week and (2) the presence of comorbid psychiatric disorders or a lifetime history of anxiety and depression at the time of infection increases the risk of developing IBS-PI. The longer duration of enteritis reflects severity of inflammation [275]. The psychosomatic disorders represent dysregulation/impairment of the central nervous system and hypothalamus-pituitary-adrenal (HPA) axis [276, 281]. While motility recordings from these patients are not available, their motility dysfunction is likely similar to that in IBS-D patients.

Take-home Messages

1. Spontaneous variations in the frequency and amplitude of GMCs from one extreme to the other in IBS-C/D patients suggest that environmental conditions (diet, stress, somatic activity) affect their regulatory mechanisms.
2. These observations speak against a genetic (mutation, polymorphism) role in motility and sensory dysfunctions in IBS. The genetic dysfunctions are stable.
3. The persistence of IBS-D-like symptoms in IBS-PI patients is likely due to epigenetic changes in genes encoding proteins of the regulatory mechanisms. Epigenetic changes in gene expression are sensitive to the cellular microenvironment.

Cellular and Molecular Mechanisms of IBS and Other Types of Constipation

Our understanding of the cellular mechanisms of motility dysfunction in functional bowel disorders (FBD) is limited, largely due to the unavailability of neuromuscular tissues from these patients and the paucity of animal models that mimic salient features of these disorders. However, clues from clinical and animal studies suggest potential cellular mechanisms. The following sections highlight the insights obtained from these studies and from recently available models of IBS-D.

Smooth Muscle and Enteric Neuronal Dysfunction

Impaired Gastrocolonic Response. Clinical studies show that the increase of motor activity—including the incidence of GMCs—in the sigmoid colon following ingestion of a meal is significantly greater in IBS-D patients than in healthy controls [22]. IBS-D patients also show an exaggerated response to exogenous CCK-8 [22]. The greater increase of GMCs after a meal in IBS-D patients associates with faster postprandial transit than in healthy subjects [259]. By contrast, the increase of postprandial colonic motor activity is significantly less in constipated patients than in healthy controls [269, 271, 282–286]. Antral distension by a balloon and duodenal instillation of lipids mimic the gastrocolonic response by increasing tone in the distal colon [287]. The increase in colonic tone by either stimulus is impaired in patients with slow-transit constipation [287].

The parasympathetic nerves mediate the gastrocolonic response to ingestion of a meal. The parasympathetic nerves synapse on nicotinic receptors on the excitatory and inhibitory motor neurons. Accumulating evidence shows that the physiologic stimulation of parasympathetic nerves by ingestion of a meal [22] or experimental electrical stimulation enhances colonic motor activity by release of ACh from excitatory cholinergic motor neurons in the myenteric plexus [42, 44, 215, 288]. Although the postprandial increase of plasma CCK after ingestion of a normal meal in healthy subjects is not enough to stimulate colonic motor activity [208], duodenal instillation of lipids and pharmacologic doses of CCK stimulate colonic motor activity [22, 208]. CCK acts on presynaptic interneurons or directly on motor neurons to release ACh and stimulate colonic contractions, while atropine blocks the contractile response to CCK in human colonic circular muscle strips [22]. Exogenous CCK stimulates GMCs in healthy volunteers as well as in IBS-D patients [22]. However, the number of GMCs stimulated by CCK is several-fold greater in IBS-D patients than in healthy controls, indicating greater and prolonged release of ACh from the cholinergic motor neurons in these patients. These findings suggest that the exaggerated motor response in IBS-D patients may be due to enhanced synthesis/release of ACh at the neuroeffector junction, slow hydrolysis of ACh at the neuromuscular junction, or sensitization of excitation-contraction coupling in circular smooth muscle cells (see Figures 10 and 11).

Findings in patients with constipation are just the opposite of those in IBS-D patients. The contractile response to ACh in circular muscle strips from idiopathic chronic constipation patients is significantly less than that in normal strips from patients with normal colon transit [289]. Interestingly, the muscle strips from constipated patients also show smaller contractile responses to electrical field stimulation (EFS). EFS induces in vitro contractions by releasing ACh from the cholinergic motor neurons. These findings suggest that the impaired colonic motor function in constipated patients is due to a reduction in the expression of ChAT, synthesis or release of ACh, or a defect in excitation-contraction coupling in circular smooth muscle cells. A decrease in the evoked release of ^{3H}choline confirms the defect in the activity of cholinergic neurons in constipated patients [290].

An impairment in excitation-contraction coupling in smooth muscle cells follows from the finding that the contractile response to edrophonium chloride—a short acting choline esterase inhibitor—is significantly lower in slow-transit constipation patients than in healthy controls [291]. ACh accumulation at the neuromuscular junction acts directly on muscarinic M_3 receptors to stimulate smooth muscle contractions. Smooth muscle dysfunction in idiopathic chronic constipation patients is evident from the inability of cathodal current to generate spikes, which suggests impairment of $Ca_v1.2b$ (L-type) calcium channels [292].

Constipated patients also display subclinical autonomic and sensory neuropathy [293, 294]. These observations may explain the hyposensitivity to colorectal distension in some constipated patients.

Abdominal Cramping/Pain. About 70% to 90% of patients with different subtypes of IBS report intermittent short-lived abdominal cramping/pain [254, 295]. The perception of pain occurs in the higher centers of the brain when they receive signals from a noxious stimulus from the periphery. Noxious signals reach the higher centers due to an unphysiological condition in the periphery, such as inflammation, amplification of a physiological signal during its transmission to the CNS (visceral hypersensitivity), or impaired supraspinal processing. IBS patients do not have any organic abnormality such as inflammation. Consequently, visceral hypersensitivity and supraspinal processing have received much attention in understanding the etiology of abdominal cramping in IBS patients.

Patients' recognition of visceral feelings—initial sensation, urge to defecate, and pain—in response to phasic or ramp distensions of a balloon in the colorectal area are used to determine the level of visceral sensitivity. Using this approach, some studies reported that about 90% of IBS patients have visceral hypersensitivity to colorectal distension [263, 296]. These investigators have proposed visceral hypersensitivity as a biomarker of IBS. However, they could not relate most symptoms of IBS to visceral hypersensitivity. They also suggested, without any scientific evidence, that visceral hypersensitivity is the source of motility dysfunction in IBS patients. The concept was that the amplified afferent signals reflexively send aberrant efferent signals to the colon to cause motility dysfunction [297–299]. In proposing these hypotheses, the investigators ignored an important fact: visceral hypersensitivity or impaired central processing does not by itself induce the sensation of pain; a peripheral signal is required.

Numerous other studies show that on average, only about 50% (range, 20% to 80% [300]) of IBS patients show visceral hypersensitivity [254, 267, 295, 301, 302]. The visceral hypersensitivity hypothesis does not explain abdominal cramping in normosensitive patients [265, 295]. In fact, none of the symptoms of IBS adequately distinguish hypersensitive from normosensitive patients [295]. This hypothesis also does not explain which reflexes alter motility function in response to visceral hypersensitivity, which alterations in colonic contractions they produce, or how the same reflexes cause diarrhea in some patients and constipation in others. This hypothesis ignores the wealth of knowledge we have about the regulation of contractions by smooth muscle cells and enteric neurons, the types of contractions they generate, and the specific functions of those contractions. Several publications have challenged this simplistic hypothesis of visceral hypersensitivity alone as the basis of IBS symptoms [300, 303].

It is noteworthy that the symptom of abdominal cramping usually follows alterations in bowel habits. In addition, repetitive high-pressure mechanical sigmoid stimulation develops hyperalgesia in normosensitive IBS patients [304–306]. GMCs that strongly compress the colon wall send afferent signals similar to those of distension of the wall by a balloon. Therefore, an increase in the frequency of GMCs could be one of the factors inducing visceral hypersensitivity.

A unifying hypothesis, based on accumulated basic science and clinical data, is that GMCs are the source of abdominal cramping. Visceral hypersensitivity, if present, worsens the sensation of abdominal cramping. Figure 37 explains the sensation of abdominal cramping with and without visceral hypersensitivity. First, the afferent signals generated by a GMC in health are below the nociceptive threshold (Figure 37A), so they do not cause the sensation of abdominal cramping. The amplitude of GMCs increases more than twofold in IBS-D patients [22]. The afferent signals they generate are noxious (Figure 37B). Each GMC may induce the sensation of abdominal cramping; however, concurrent visceral hypersensitivity will exaggerate the pain [295, 301]. Figure 37C shows a scenario in which abdominal cramping is entirely due to visceral hypersensitivity. In this case, a GMC of normal or below-normal amplitude will induce the sensation of cramping. The intensity of pain will relate to the degree of hypersensitivity.

There is no evidence that the nociceptive threshold decreases to levels where the afferent signals generated by RPCs become noxious. Were this to happen, patients would feel a continuous sensation of pain, because RPCs are always present somewhere in the colon. By contrast, GMCs occur only a limited number of times per day, even in IBS patients who have more. Therefore, abdominal cramping occurs intermittently and only for the duration of a GMC.

Figure 37D illustrates another scenario in which abdominal cramping may occur with or without visceral hypersensitivity. Impairment of descending inhibition prevents relaxation of the receiving segment ahead of it. Receptive relaxation decreases in some IBS patients [247]. In this situation, the afferent signals due to ballooning of the receiving segment will add to those of the GMCs to become a noxious signal. This is likely to happen when impairment of descending inhibition prevents relaxation of the internal anal sphincter as the GMC is attempting to push feces through for defecation or when voluntary relaxation of the puborectalis muscle and the external

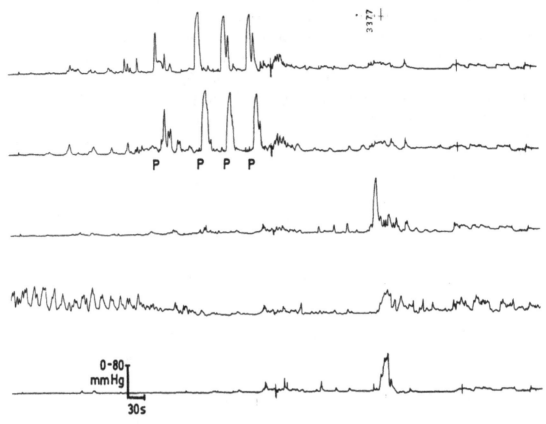

FIGURE 42: GMCs in the ascending colon of a severely constipated patient. Each GMC induced a discrete sensation of pain. The recording ports were 12 cm apart. According to the authors, a kink in the manometric tube located distal to the bottom port stimulated these GMCs. The amplitude of these GMCs are within the normal range. On a speculative note, pain might have resulted from hypersensitivity in the ascending colon, distension of colon segment due to GMC attempting to push fecal material past compacted stool (see Fig. 37D) due to obstruction from compacted stool and impaired descending inhibition. (Reproduced with permission from Bassotti G et al., *Gut*, 29: 1173–1179, 1988 [203].)

sphincter are impaired. Another potential scenario is when a GMC attempts to push fecal material past compacted stool in constipated patients (Figure 42).

Take-home Messages

1. About 90% of IBS patients report intermittent short-lived abdominal cramping. However, only about 50% of these patients have visceral hypersensitivity.
2. Visceral hypersensitivity does not correlate well with most symptoms of IBS.

3. GMC is the stimulus from the periphery that sends perceptible signals to the CNS. At higher amplitudes of GMCs, these signals are noxious and produce the sensation of abdominal cramping/pain that lasts for the total duration of a GMC.

4. Concurrent visceral hypersensitivity and/or failure of descending relaxation enhance the afferent signals generated by a GMC. When this happens, normal-amplitude GMCs produce the sensation of cramping/pain.

5. The frequency of GMCs relates to the symptoms of diarrhea and constipation in IBS patients. A significant increase in GMC frequency causes diarrhea, while a significant decrease causes constipation.

6. The frequency of GMCs may serve as a biomarker of IBS subtypes.

Stress. Stress is an adaptive physiological response of living systems to real or perceived life-threatening situations. This response begins in the CNS. The release of corticotrophin-releasing hormone (CRH) from the paraventricular nucleus of the hypothalamus is an early and essential step in the stress response [307]. The central release of CRH and other mediators, such as arginine vasopressin (AVP), stimulate the neuroendocrine system comprised of autonomic neurons and the HPA axis, which modulate the adaptive and maladaptive responses of peripheral organs in a stress- and cell-type-specific manner. Nontranscriptional mechanisms largely mediate the immediate and short-term effects of acute stress. For example, acute stress releases norepinephrine in the amygdala and hypothalamus to sharpen focus and attention [308]. It also increases the heart rate and blood flow in preparation for the "fight-or-flight" response [309].

The HPA axis and the sympathetic nervous system show subtle alterations in IBS patients in the resting state and after stressors [310–321]. Acute psychological as well as physical stress modestly stimulate colonic motor activity. Animal studies show that hypothalamic release of CRH and vagal nerves mediate the stimulation of colonic motor function by acute stress [322–324].

Acute stress modestly reduces the thresholds to colorectal distension in IBS patients relative to normal subjects, presumably due to baseline alterations in the HPA axis and the autonomic nervous system [310, 325, 326]. However, we do not know the cause-and-effect relationship between individual mediators of stress and transient sensitization of visceral afferents.

The effects of acute stress are transient, lasting more or less for the duration of the stressor. Clinical studies show that chronic stress, as opposed to acute stress, precipitates/relapses or exacerbates the symptoms of IBS [327, 328]. This is not surprising, because stress targets some of the same physiological functions already impaired in IBS patients, i.e., altered motor function and visceral hypersensitivity to motor events in the colon.

The mechanisms by which chronic stress relapses or exaggerates the symptoms of IBS are not investigable in patients due to ethical considerations and lack of availability of neuromuscular tissues. Animal studies show that heterotypic or homotypic intermittent chronic stress (HeICS and

HoICS, respectively) induces visceral hypersensitivity in rats that persists after the stress is over by the following mechanisms [329, 330] (Figure 43).

1. Chronic stress releases CRH and angiotensin vasopressin from the paraventricular nucleus in the hypothalamus.
2. CRH and arginine vasopressin stimulate the locus ceruleus/norepinephrine system. In par-

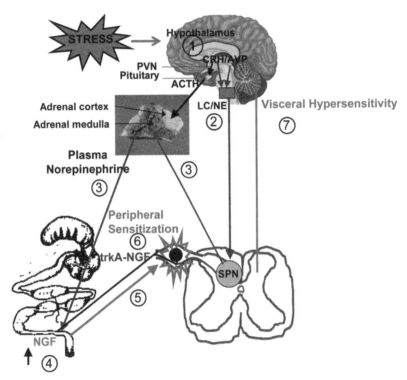

FIGURE 43: Cartoon showing the mechanisms of HeICS-induced visceral hypersensitivity to colorectal distension (CRD) in relation to the well-established elements of the stress response. **Step 1:** Stress releases CRH and angiotensin vasopressin from the paraventricular nucleus in the hypothalamus. CRH releases adrenocorticotropic hormone and other mediators from the pituitary. **Step 2:** CRH and arginine vasopressin stimulate the locus ceruleus/norepinephrine system. **Step 3:** Activation of the sympathetic preganglionic neurons releases norepinephrine/epinephrine in blood stream from the adrenal medulla. **Step 4:** Norepinephrine elevates the expression of NGF in colonic muscularis externa and mucosa/submucosa. **Step 5:** NGF complexes with trkA receptors, and the complex transports retrograde to the thoracolumbar DRG. **Step 6:** NGF/trkA complex sensitizes colon-specific neurons by modulating the expression and characteristics of ion channels **Step 7:** The amplification of afferent signal in response to CRD is perceived as abdominal pain/discomfort.

allel, CRH releases adrenocorticotropic hormone from the pituitary, which releases corticosterone from the adrenal cortex.

3. Activation of the greater splanchnic sympathetic preganglionic neurons releases norepinephrine from the chromaffin cells in the adrenal medulla into the blood stream [331, 332]. The increase in plasma norepinephrine persists for several hours [333].

4. Norepinephrine enhances the expression of NGF in the colon wall.

5. NGF complexes with trkA receptors, and the complex transports retrograde to the thoracolumbar DRG [334].

6. NGF/trkA complex in the DRG sensitizes the ion channels.

7. Hypersensitization of these ion channels amplifies the afferent signals in response to colonic distension/compression to increase perception. This sensitization occurs in the absence of a detectable inflammatory response in the muscularis externa or in the mucosa/submucosa.

Based on the topology and phenotypes of afferent nerve endings in the colon wall [245–247, 335, 336], an increase in NGF in the muscularis externa mediates the induction of visceral hypersensitivity by HeICS, whereas an increase in NGF in the mucosa/submucosa mediates an altered physiological response to digesta in the lumen.

The systemic upregulation of norepinephrine by HeICS also enhances the reactivity of colonic circular smooth muscle cells to ACh in muscle strips as well as in single isolated cells, resulting in an increase in colonic transit and pellet defecation, producing diarrhealike conditions in rats [333] (Figure 44). Adrenalectomy, but not the depletion of sympathetic neurons by guanethidine, blocks these effects. Corticosterone, CRH, or vagal nerves do not mediate these effects.

Norepinephrine enhances expression of the pore-forming $\alpha_{1C}1b$ subunit of $Ca_v1.2b$ channels in circular smooth muscle cells, which increases Ca^{2+} influx in response to ACh [173] (see Figure 11) to enhance the amplitude of contractions and hence colonic transit. These effects peak at about 8 hours after the last stressor and return to baseline by 24 hours [333]. These findings show that prolonged upregulation of plasma norepinephrine by chronic stress remodels the cellular regulatory mechanisms, resulting in organ dysfunction. Similar remodeling occurs in CNS neurons and cardiac muscle cells [337–340]. Acute chronic stress does not induce these effects. By contrast, HoICS induces hyperalgesia in rats that lasts up to 40 days [330]. The prolonged effects of chronic stress in animal models is consistent with clinical observations that the symptoms of IBS improve with the resolution of major life stressors.

Take-home Messages

1. Chronic, rather than acute, stress in animal models produces prolonged motor dysfunction and visceral hypersensitivity.

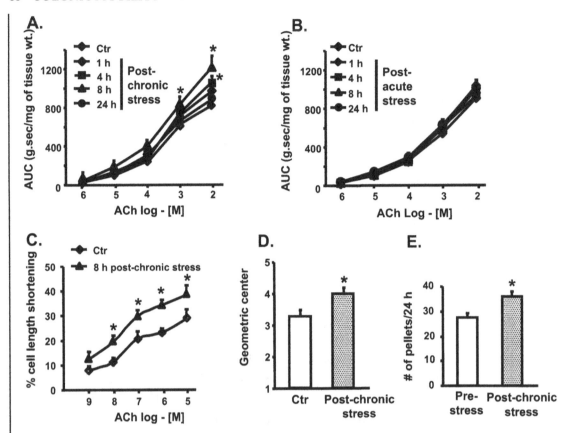

FIGURE 44: Effects of HeICS on colonic smooth muscle contractility and motor function. (A) The contractile response to ACh in colonic circular muscle strips increased significantly at 4 hours and 8 hours after 9-day heterotypic intermittent chronic stress protocol but returned to baseline after 24 hours. (B) The contractile response to ACh did not change 1 hour, 4 hours, 8 hours, or 24 hours after 1-day acute stress protocol. (C) The cell shortening to ACh increased significantly in single dispersed smooth muscle cells obtained 8 hours after 9-day HeICS protocol, when compared to that in single cells from age-matched sham-treated controls. (D) The colonic transit (measured as geometric center) was significantly greater 8 hours after 9-day HeICS protocol, when compared with sham-treated age-matched controls. (E) The number of fecal pellets/24 hours significantly increased after 9-day HeICS protocol. *p < 0.05 vs. age-matched sham-treated controls. AUC = area under contractions, Ctr = controls.

2. Chronic stress precipitates/exaggerates the symptoms of IBS.
3. Sustained increase in plasma norepinephrine following chronic stress makes a major contribution to the development of visceral hypersensitivity and altered motor function.
4. Increase in the expression of NGF in the colonic muscularis externa mediates the induction of visceral hypersensitivity by norepinephrine.
5. The retrograde transport of NGF/trkA complex sensitizes the colon-specific DRG neurons.

Early-Life Trauma and IBS

Retrospective studies show that prenatal, infant, or childhood trauma predisposes to developing the symptoms of IBS at an early age, which continue in adulthood [341–350]. Animal models of neonatal trauma support the hypothesis that early-life trauma results in visceral hypersensitivity to colorectal distension and/or motility dysfunction in adulthood.

Mechanical or chemical irritation in neonates results in persistent sensitization of the spinal afferents and visceral hypersensitivity to colorectal distension in adulthood [351]. Maternal separation of neonatal rats induces allodynia and hyperalgesia in adulthood by enhancing expression of NGF in the colon wall [352, 353]. In this model, the proliferation and degranulation of mast cells increase the expression of NGF, which mediates hypersensitivity to colorectal distension. The maternally separated rats also show heightened response to acute water avoidance stress.

A randomized double-blind placebo-controlled study found little improvement in symptoms of IBS- PI patients by prednisone treatment [354]. Therefore, it is not clear whether neonatal maternal separation represents a model of IBS or IBD. Regardless, we do not know yet the epigenetic mechanisms, described later, that underlie colonic motor dysfunction and visceral hypersensitivity in response to adverse early life experiences.

Neonatal inflammation on postnatal day 10 (PND 10) significantly enhances the mRNA and protein expression of the α_{1C}-subunit of $Ca_v1.2$ (L-type) calcium channels, $G\alpha_q$, and the regulatory myosin light chain kinase (RLC_{20}) in adulthood [355]. The enhanced expression of each of these cell-signaling proteins favors increased reactivity to ACh (see Figure 11). As a result, the contractile responses of single smooth muscle cells and of circular smooth muscle strips from affected rats are greater than those from control rats. The faster colonic transit and greater pellet output in these rats simulate the diarrhealike conditions of IBS-D patients.

The neonatal insult in these rats also enhances the VIP content of muscularis externa and plasma concentrations of norepinephrine. The motility dysfunction in adult rats who received neonatal inflammatory insult occurs in the absence of any inflammation or structural damage. Of note, a similar inflammatory insult in adult rats does not result in enhancement of smooth muscle reactivity to ACh or faster colonic transit [355].

Note that there is seldom a perfect animal model of human disease. However, these models closely mimic specific features of IBS and their regulatory mechanisms. They are indispensable in identifying the underlying mechanisms of organ dysfunction, allowing for testing of hypotheses in humans and development of therapeutic agents.

Take-home Messages

1. Neonatal psychological and inflammatory insults induce visceral hypersensitivity and motor dysfunction in adulthood.
2. The maladaptive effects of chronic stress on gut function—altered motor function and visceral hypersensitivity to motor events in the colon—are the same as those that characterize IBS patients. However, the mechanisms by which chronic stress exaggerates these effects in IBS patients may be different from those that underlie abnormal functions without stress.

Impaired Enteric Reflexes

Balloon distension in in vitro experiments in the intact human colon stimulates contractions above and relaxation below it [47]. The ascending stimulation—mediated by the release of ACh—is blunted in the colon of slow-transit patients [287], which agrees with other findings that the synthesis and/or release of ACh and the excitation-contraction coupling are impaired in constipated patients. However, the descending relaxation—mediated by NO—is not different between slow-transit constipation patients and healthy controls, suggesting a normal function of inhibitory motor neurons. In vitro findings in muscle strips from patients with idiopathic chronic constipation support the notion that their nitrergic neurons are functioning near normal [292]. The normality of inhibitory neuronal function, however, may not be universal in constipation. One study found enhanced NO-induced and ATP-induced relaxation in a group of idiopathic chronic constipation patients [289].

Take-home Message

Impaired release of ACh proximal to the site of balloon distension confirms the defects in the synthesis/release of ACh and/or excitation-contraction coupling in smooth muscle cells in slow-transit patients.

Impaired Smooth Muscle Excitation-Contraction Coupling in Slow-Transit Constipation

The prevalence and severity of slow-transit constipation are higher in females than in males [356, 357]. Alterations in cell-signaling proteins of excitation-contraction coupling in smooth muscle cells in response to progesterone partly explain this disparity. Progesterone acting on its nuclear receptors regulates the expression of some G proteins ($G\alpha_q$ and $G\alpha_{i3}$) negatively and others ($G\alpha_s$)

positively [358–360]. Progesterone levels in females with slow-transit constipation are normal. However, due to genetic/epigenetic abnormality, these patients overexpress progesterone B (PGR-B) receptors on colonic smooth muscle cells. As a result, transcription and protein expression of $G\alpha_q$ decrease, while those of $G\alpha_s$ increase. The suppression of $G\alpha_q$ reduces the binding of ligands such as ACh and CCK to their respective receptors coupled with this G protein, resulting in reduction in smooth muscle contractility in response to ligands (Figure 45). The contractile response to diacylglycerol and KCl, which bypass the $G\alpha_q$ protein, remains intact, indicating normality of the rest of excitation-contraction coupling (see Figure 11). Incidentally, progesterone concurrently suppresses the expression of COX-1 and enhances that of COX-2 [359], decreasing the generation of thromboxane A_2 (TxA_2) and prostaglandin F2α ($PGF_2\alpha$) and increasing the expression of prostaglandin E_2 (PGE_2). $PGF_2\alpha$ and TxA_2 contract smooth muscle cells, while PGE_2 inhibits these contractions. However, the contribution of these pathways in spontaneous colonic motor function is unknown.

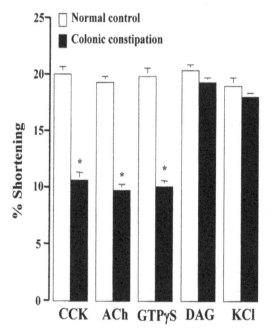

FIGURE 45: The shortening of single isolated smooth muscle cells obtained from normal controls and from patients with chronic constipation. The cell shortening in response to agonists CCK, ACh, and GTPγS was smaller in tissues from constipated patients than in those from control subjects. By contrast, cell shortening in response to agonists that bypass the receptors and G proteins—diacylglycerol and KCl—does not differ between tissues from constipated patients and controls. These data show impairment of specific components of cell-signaling proteins of excitation-contraction coupling in smooth muscle cells from constipated patients. (Reproduced with permission from Xiao et al. and Behar, J, *Gastroenterology*, 128: 667–675, 2005 [358].)

Take-home Message

Upregulation of progesterone B receptors in smooth muscle cells in the human colon explain the higher incidence of slow-transit constipation in female patients.

Role of ICCs

Some reports found a deficiency in the volume of ICC throughout the colon of patients with slow-transit constipation [99, 361–364]. However, these publications did not establish a cause-and-effect relationship between the reduction in the volume of ICC and patient symptoms, disorders in colonic motor activity, or its regulatory mechanisms. According to numerous clinical studies cited above, the slow transit in these patients is primarily due to the reduction in GMCs. There is no evidence that ICC regulate GMCs, which occur independently of slow waves. A recent study has demonstrated that ICC do not mediate the neuronal input to smooth muscle cells [365]. The normal function of inhibitory nitrergic motor neurons in descending inhibition is additional evidence that reduction in the volume of ICC in constipated patients does not mediate neuronal input to smooth muscle cells [79, 365]. The RPCs regulated by slow waves play a relatively smaller role in slow-transit constipation. However, the slow waves do not show a defect in in vitro recordings from the colonic smooth muscle cells of slow-transit patients [292]. The slow-wave frequency and its spatial organization are not different between IBS patients and healthy controls under resting conditions and after stimulation with a meal or neostigmine [366].

Take-home Messages

1. The volume of ICC is decreased in the colon of slow-transit constipation patients. However, there is no evidence that this decrease causes motility dysfunction or visceral hypersensitivity.
2. Both the frequency of slow waves and nitrergic neuronal function are normal in these patients.

Role of Alterations in the Expression of Neuropeptides in the Myenteric Plexus and Structural Damage to Enteric Neurons and Smooth Muscle Cells

Several immunohistochemical, radioimmunoassay, and ultrastructural studies have identified abnormalities in enteric neurons and smooth muscle cells in tissue from IBS patients [367–374]. Most of these studies are on tissues obtained from severely constipated patients undergoing colonic resection. Disappointingly, these findings are often divergent; some show a positive change, some show a negative one, and others find no change in the same parameter, such as damage to neurons containing a certain neurotransmitter or global damage to neurons [357]. This is partly due to the qualitative nature of analysis in these methods and the heterogeneity of tissues and observations at the microscopic level. Another major limitation is the absence of efforts to establish a cause-and-effect relationship between the findings and functional impairment. These approaches have been very helpful in identifying the cause of a disease when the defect is simple and confined to one type of cell, such as aganglionosis in Hirschsprung's disease. However, these approaches seem to be of limited use in complex diseases like IBS.

Epigenetic Dysregulation

Over the past three decades, discoveries of gene mutations that cause or contribute to simple Mendelian diseases, such as sickle cell anemia, hemophilia, and cystic fibrosis have been reported [375–377]. However, the search for gene mutation that causes complex diseases, such as diabetes, most cancers, asthma, inflammatory bowel disease, and functional bowel disorders has largely been unsuccessful. Complex diseases exhibit an inheritable component but do not follow Mendel's laws. For example, discordance of monozygotic twins reaches 30%–50% in diabetes, 70% in multiple sclerosis and rheumatoid arthritis, and 80% in breast cancer [378]. Differential environmental factors during fetal and neonatal development usually account for discordance of monozygotic twins. The simple diseases following Mendel's laws begin predominantly before puberty [379], whereas complex diseases tend to appear later in life and may exhibit more than one peak of increased risk of onset [380]. The simple diseases progressively worsen after onset, whereas complex diseases, such as major psychosis, inflammatory bowel disease, functional bowel disorders, and rheumatoid arthritis, exhibit relapses and remissions. Epigenetics plays a prominent role in cancer and autoimmune and inflammatory diseases [381–386].

The inherited genetic code is identical in all cell types in an organism, with the exception of a few, such as the gametes [387]. During ontogeny, epigenetic mechanisms set the transcription rates of each gene in the genome ranging from complete silence to full activation, imparting phenotype to each cell. The transcription rates of different genes are set for survival of the fetus and the neonate as well as for optimal responses of the cells to their microenvironment of hormones, neurotransmitters, growth factors, and inflammatory mediators in adulthood. However, if the fetus (indirectly through the mother) or the neonate is exposed to psychological or inflammatory stress, the transcription rates of genes vulnerable at the time of insult may be set at abnormal levels, ensuring current survival but leading to abnormal cell function in adulthood, causing a complex disease. This is known as Barker's hypothesis [388] or neonatal/fetal programming.

Epigenetic regulation during neonatal inflammatory or psychological stress can modify gene expression by post-transcriptional histone modifications and by DNA methylation.

Posttranslational Histone Modifications. DNA is packaged tightly into a highly organized and dynamic protein-DNA complex called chromatin. The basic subunit of chromatin is the nucleosome, which contains about 146 bp of DNA wrapped twice around an octomer core of four histones (two molecules each of histones H2A, H2B, H3, and H4) in a 1.65 left-handed superhelical turn [389–392] (Figure 46).

Normally, the histone proteins are positively charged and form tight electrostatic associations with negatively charged DNA, which results in tight compaction of chromatin and inaccessibility of the DNA to transcription factors and transcriptional machinery. The N-terminal tails are the main sites of posttranslational modifications including acetylation, methylation, phosphorylation, citrullination, sumoylation, ubiquitination, and ADP-ribosylation by enzymes, and this affects their function in gene regulation [393]. Acetylation, one of the most widespread modifications of histone proteins, including H2B, H3, and H4, occurs on lysine residues in the N-terminal tail and on the surface of the nucleosome core as part of gene regulation [394]. The addition of an acetyl group

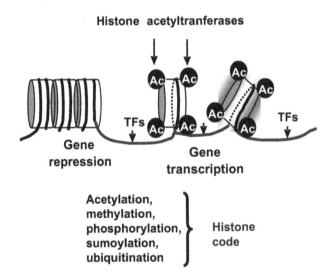

FIGURE 46: Nucleosome is the smallest unit of chromatin. On the left, the packing of the first few nucleosomes is tight so that the transcription factors do not have access to the DNA wrapped around these nucleosomes. Acetylation of the N-terminal histone protein tails by a histone acetyltransferase reduces its positive charge to form a more relaxed configuration with DNA, which allows the transcription factors and transcriptional machinery access to their recognition sites on the promoters of specific genes to induce transcription.

to histone proteins reduces their positive charge to form a more relaxed configuration with DNA, which allows the transcription factors and transcriptional machinery access to their recognition sites on the promoters of specific genes to induce transcription.

The opposing actions of histone acetyltransferases (HATs) and histone deacetylases (HDACs) control the acetyl group turnover. The HATs are present as part of large protein complexes and act as transcriptional coactivators. The deacetylases (HDACs) are recruited to target genes via their direct association with transcriptional activators and repressors, as well as their incorporation into large multiprotein transcriptional complexes [383]. Together, these two classes of enzymes account for the coordinated changes in chromatin structure that carry out its functions [395, 396]. The balance between the actions of these enzymes is a key regulatory mechanism for gene expression and governs numerous developmental processes and disease states [383]. Lysine acetylation is associated with active gene expression and open chromatin. H3K9ac and H4K16ac are two histone modifications often associated with euchromatin. Chromatin immunoprecipitation (ChIP) assay shows that neonatal colonic inflammation significantly increases the association of RNA polymerase II (RNAP II) with the core promoter region of the *Cacna1c* gene in adulthood, which would increase the transcription rate of this gene (Figure 47).

Methylation of lysine and arginine residues can occur in histones H3 and H4, in the mono-, di-, or tri-methylated form [397]. Depending on the site and type of histone, the methylation pattern will result in a different transcriptional outcome. Methylation of H3K9, H3K27, and H4K20 links generally to heterochromatin formation, whereas methylation of H3K4 and H3K36 associates with transcriptionally active regions. Di- and tri-methylation of histone H3 lysine 4 (H3K4me2 and H3K4me3) are hallmarks of chromatin at active genes [398].

DNA Methylation. Covalent addition of methyl groups, catalyzed by enzymes known as DNA methyltransferases (DNMTs), modifies DNA to alter gene transcription. DNA methylation occurs at specific dinucleotide sites along the genome, cytosines 5' of guanines (CpG sites). About 40% to 50% of the protein-coding genes have GC-rich sequences in their promoter regions, known as CpG islands, and about 70% to 80% of all CpG dinucleotides in the genome are methylated [399]. DNA methylation affects the correct temporal and spatial silencing of gene expression during development and during disease processes such as tumor progression [400]. The methylation of CpG islands restricts the access of transcription factors to the promoter region, thereby suppressing transcription of the targeted genes [401].

Four members of DNA methylation transferases (DNMTs) regulate DNA methylation in mammals. DNMT1 has a high affinity for the hemimethylated form of DNA, maintaining the constitutive methylation status of the DNA [402]. DNMT2 does not have a DNA-binding domain, and its role in DNA methylation is unknown [403]. By contrast, the roles of DNMT3a and

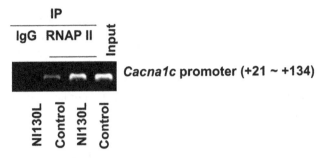

FIGURE 47: RNAP II interaction with the *Cacna1c* core promoter is markedly elevated in the colonic muscularis externa of adult rats subjected to neonatal inflammation. Freshly obtained full-thickness rat colon tissues were immersed in warm, carbogenated Krebs solution with 5% O_2/95% CO_2 mix. The mucosal/submucosal layers were removed. Muscle strips were cut along circumferential axis and snap-frozen in liquid nitrogen. Frozen tissues were pulverized in liquid nitrogen, and chromatin immunoprecipitation (ChIP) assay was performed using ChIP-IT^{TM} Express Enzymatic kit (Active Motif, Carlsbad, CA). RNA polymerase II (RNAP II) mouse monoclonal antibody and mouse IgG (negative control) were used to precipitate RNAP II–bound DNA fragments from sheared chromatins. 10% sheared chromatin served as input control. Polymerase chain reaction (PCR) was performed by using *Cacna1c*-specific primers and Platinum Taq DNA Polymerase. PCR products were subjected to electrophoresis on 2% agarose gels, stained with ethidium bromide.

DNMT3b in regulating DNA methylation in oncogenesis and in response to stressors are well established [402].

Genetics

Functional bowel disorders do not have the traits of genetic diseases. Genetic alterations (mutations and polymorphisms) inherited from parents or mutations due to environmental factors once acquired are irreversible. Mutations in a gene may produce a wrong protein or no protein at all; polymorphisms may produce a variant protein. The functional effects of mutations and polymorphisms are stable.

By contrast, the severity and types of symptoms in functional bowel disorders vary, arguing against a genetic component [404, 405]. The symptoms of altered bowel function in IBS-C/D patients switch from one extreme to the other. Acute events such as stress precipitate/exaggerate the symptoms of functional bowel disorders [328]. All these characteristics of functional bowel disorders suggest fluctuating expression of proteins causing dysfunction, a result of epigenetic regulation rather than genetic variance. Epigenetic mechanisms, discussed above, can alter the expression of target proteins in target cells, such as smooth muscle cells and afferent neurons, in response to changes in their microenvironment.

Take-home Messages

1. Epigenetic regulation modifies the expression of selective genes in cells following changes in their microenvironment.
2. If the changes in microenvironment occur during the vulnerable stages of fetal and neonatal development, the changes in expressions of selective genes may persist into adulthood to cause complex diseases, such as IBS.
3. The relapsing/recurring changes in symptoms of IBS do not make them candidates for genetic mutations/polymorphisms.

INFLAMMATORY BOWEL DISEASE

Inflammatory bowel disease (IBD), comprised of ulcerative colitis and Crohn's disease, is a chronic, idiopathic, and relapsing inflammation of the gut. Ulcerative colitis usually begins in the rectum/distal colon and progresses orally. Crohn's disease usually begins in the terminal ileum but may extend to other areas of the gastrointestinal tract, especially the colon (Crohn's colitis). The two types of IBD are clinically, immunologically, and morphologically distinct. In spite of differing etiologies, the primary symptoms of both types of IBD (diarrhea, abdominal cramping, and urgency of defecation) are strikingly similar. Stools of ulcerative colitis patients are bloody and contain mucus.

IBD patients present with motor diarrhea (*diarrhee motrice*), frequent nonwatery stools [406]. The daily frequency of unformed stools is about five times per day in mild to moderate pancolitis and four times per day in mild to moderate distal colitis. These numbers increase with severity of colitis. About 80% to 90% of pancolitis patients show urgency and nocturnal defecation, and 30% have incontinence [407]. About 80% of these patients report incomplete evacuation. Paradoxically, about 20% to 30% of pancolitis and distal colitis patients pass hard stools [407]. The total gut transit in ulcerative colitis patients is not different from that in healthy controls [408]. However, the proximal colon shows stasis while the rectosigmoid colon shows rapid propulsion, which counteract each other to produce normal whole colon transit [409–412].

Motility Dysfunction in Colonic Inflammation

Limited data are available from manometric recordings in ulcerative colitis patients due to the risk of perforation; much less is available from Crohn's colitis patients. However, the disturbances in small intestinal motor activity in Crohn's disease are similar to those seen in the colon of ulcerative colitis patients [413]. Much of our understanding of motility dysfunction in both types of IBD has come from animal models of inflammation.

Studies in IBD patients and in experimental models show that inflammation suppresses RPCs and tonic contractions, at the same time enhancing the frequency of GMCs [19, 166, 409,

414–416]. The degree of suppression of RPCs and increase in the frequency of GMCs are independent variables, but each correlates with the intensity of inflammation and clinical symptoms [166, 409]. The stimulation of GMCs and suppression of RPCs are most intense in the inflamed part of the colon. However, inflammation in one part of a gut organ can reflexively alter motility function at distal locations [417], which means that colitis in the distal colon may suppress RPCs in the middle and the proximal colon.

The above motility dysfunctions explain most of the observed clinical symptoms in IBD patients.

Note that most studies of ulcerative colitis have recruited patients with mild to moderate colitis. Patients with severe colitis are likely to have more intense motility dysfunction, as judged by inflammation in experimental models.

In one group of patients with moderate colitis, the frequency of GMCs increased about two-fold over that in healthy controls [39]. The increased frequency of GMCs produces frequent mass movements. The concurrent suppression of RPCs facilitates distal propulsion of luminal contents. The GMCs that propagate up to the rectum or the distal sigmoid colon stimulate afferent signals to generate urges to defecate as well as causing descending relaxation of the internal anal sphincter in preparation for defecation. A strong GMC propagating to the rectum can result in involuntary defecation (fecal incontinence). It is noteworthy that even though the frequency of GMCs increases in colonic inflammation, it still occurs no more than 10 to 15 times per day in moderate colitis. The frequent rapid propulsion by GMCs reduces the contact time of fecal material with the inflamed mucosa to reduce absorption of water and electrolytes. In addition, the concurrent suppression of RPCs reduces the mixing and turning over of fecal material to reduce its total exposure to the mucosa. Together, these two factors result in unformed, but not watery, stools. Note that the degree of stool softness depends on the intensity of inflammation, which stimulates GMCs and suppresses RPCs.

The GMCs compress the colon wall very strongly because of their large amplitudes (>100 mm Hg). Excessive occurrence of GMCs causes hemorrhages, thick mucus secretion, and mucosal erosions in experimental models [418]. These lesions explain the bloody stools with mucus characteristic of ulcerative colitis. While the GMCs are also the driving force for diarrhea in IBS-D patients, their mucosa is not inflamed and fragile as in ulcerative colitis patients. So while IBS-D patients have diarrhea, they do not have bloody stools. The higher frequency of GMCs propagating up to the rectum in the inflamed colon induces frequent bowel movements in ulcerative colitis patients (motor diarrhea).

In a canine model of moderately severe acute pancolitis, the frequency of GMCs increased more than 10-fold [166]. About half of these GMCs propagated to the sigmoid colon, resulting in uncontrollable defecation (urgency). The rest occasionally expelled gas and caused tenesmus, which may result if a GMC generates the urge to defecate in the absence of any stool in the rectum. The false urges caused by GMCs in an empty distal colon may also generate the sensation of incomplete evacuation. These symptoms and abnormal motility cease on recovery from inflammation.

About 20% of ulcerative colitis patients pass hard stools [407], giving the perception that they are constipated. The ascending colon in colitis patients shows stasis, while the sigmoid colon shows rapid transit [408]. Concurrent manometric recordings from the ascending and sigmoid colons of these patients are not available. However, on a speculative note, stasis in the ascending may result if inflammation in the sigmoid colon reflexively suppresses both RPCs and GMCs in the proximal colon, thus prolonging stool transit and forming hard stools. However, when these hard stools reach the inflamed sigmoid colon, the frequently occurring GMCs propel them rapidly, so that the passing of hard stools gives the impression of constipation.

One study in patients with inactive Crohn's ileitis reported suppression of small intestinal RPCs and stimulation of GMCs [413]. These effects are similar to the colonic motor dysfunction seen in ulcerative colitis patients. Animal models of ileal inflammation confirm these findings [419]. Ileal inflammation suppresses RPCs in the ileum as well as proximal to it, extending up to the stomach. Many of the GMCs stimulated by ileal inflammation propagate up to the terminal ileum. The animals are visibly uncomfortable during the passage of an ileal GMC. The frequency of bowel movements increases several-fold due to ileal inflammation [419]. Spontaneous GMCs in the ileum occur primarily in the interdigestive state [6]. However, in ileal inflammation, they also occur after a meal, resulting in rapid emptying of undigested food and bile from the ileum into the colon.

The increase in the incidence of GMCs in the ileum, by itself, cannot induce frequent defecation. Colon involvement is necessary. Animal studies show that many GMCs originating in the ileum propagate to the colon, causing uncontrollable defecation if they propagate to the sigmoid colon [420]. Furthermore, postprandial GMCs occurring during ileal inflammation rapidly transfer undigested chyme into the colon, which increases its osmotic load to suppress RPCs and stimulate colonic GMCs [149]. In an animal model of ileal inflammation, a collection cannula located distal to the inflamed segment of the ileum collected copious discharge of mucus with fresh blood [419]. These data indicate that an excessively high incidence of GMCs in the inflamed ileum likely causes the severe hemorrhage seen in some Crohn's disease patients [421, 422].

Take-home Messages

1. Increase in the frequency of GMCs and suppression of RPCs characterize colonic motor dysfunction in IBD patients.

2. Frequent mass movements by GMCs cause diarrhea and urgency.

3. A difference between IBS-D and IBD patients is that RPCs are suppressed in IBD patients but not in IBS-D patients.

4. Strong compression of the colon wall with inflamed mucosa by GMCs causes hemorrhage. Hemorrhage does not occur in IBS-D patients because their mucosa is not fragile.

Visceral Hypersensitivity in IBD

The sensation of pain in IBD patients is generally located in the lower abdomen and rectal areas. Most information on visceral hypersensitivity in these patients comes from distension studies in the rectum. There are two schools of thought regarding rectal hypersensitivity in IBD patients. One is that the rectum is hypersensitive to balloon distension in patients with moderate colitis, when compared with healthy subjects or patients in remission [408, 414, 423]. These patients present with diarrhea, urgency, feeling of incomplete evacuation, tenesmus, incontinence, and intermittent lower abdominal pain. The rectum in patients with active colitis is less compliant than in controls or in quiescent colitis. The other school of thought is that the rectum is hyposensitive in mild or inactive ulcerative colitis or when active inflammation is in the ileum (Crohn's disease) [424, 425]. Data from distension studies in the sigmoid colon are not available.

The visceral hypersensitivity that accompanies inflammation is due to the upregulation of neurotrophin growth factor (NGF) in response to the enhanced production of inflammatory mediators in the colon wall [426, 427]. Animal models of inflammation show consistent visceral hypersensitivity, which subsides after inflammation is over [428–432].

Rectal hypersensitivity in moderate to severe inflammation explains the frequent urge to defecate in response to the arrival of smaller volumes of feces in the rectum. The descending inhibition of the internal anal sphincter in response to rectal distension remains intact in colitis patients [408], suggesting that the internal anal sphincter does not obstruct the mass propulsion by a propagating GMC preceding defecation. The perception of pain in these patients is therefore entirely due to strong compression of the colon wall and sensitization of the afferent splanchnic neurons. Colitis patients in remission are relatively free of symptoms because the events precipitating them—excessive frequency of GMCs—are absent. This may happen regardless of whether the afferent sensitization normalizes during remission.

Take-home Messages

1. Strong compression of the sigmoid colon along with visceral hypersensitivity causes the sensation of intermittent short-lived pain in IBD patients.

2. Increased expression of NGF in the colon wall mediates visceral hypersensitivity in animal models of colonic inflammation.

Cellular and Molecular Mechanisms

A great deal of our understanding of the cellular mechanisms of motility dysfunction in colonic inflammation has come from animal models of inflammation [433]. The animal models of IBD fairly well replicate the acute inflammatory component of human disease; however, they lack the remission and relapse features. While the animal models have these limitations, they have the advantage of having more or less similar lesions within the study group, and they are free of disease modification by medications. In many cases, the animals serve as their own controls.

Smooth Muscle Dysfunction

Organ bath studies show that circular smooth muscle tissues from human ulcerative colitis [434, 435], Crohn's disease [436], and their animal models [12, 17, 437–439] are less reactive to ACh than the tissue from respective controls. ACh acts directly on muscarinic M_3 receptors on smooth muscle cells to stimulate contractions. Therefore, the suppression of contractility in inflammation is due, in part, to a defect in the excitation-contraction coupling in smooth muscle cells. Studies in human tissue from ulcerative colitis patients [440] show little change in the characteristics of slow waves. The nitrergic nerves also seem to function normally in tissue from ulcerative colitis patients, which concurs with normal relaxation of the anal sphincter in response to rectal distension [408].

A major abnormality contributing to the suppression of contractility by inflammation seems to be in the excitation-contraction coupling in smooth muscle cells. TNFα and IL-1β, prominent inflammatory mediators, significantly suppress expression of the pore-forming α_{1C}-subunit of $Ca_v 1.2b$ (L-type) calcium channels in human and animal colonic circular smooth muscle cells [62, 177, 441–443]. These inflammatory mediators activate NF-κB, which translocates to the nucleus to suppress transcription of the gene encoding the α_{1C}-subunit. The suppression of the α_{1C}-subunit reduces the number of calcium channels in smooth muscle membrane and the calcium influx/inward calcium current moving through them [62, 173]. The inhibition of NF-κB activation, in vivo or in vitro, blocks the suppression of $Ca_v 1.2$ channels to restore cell contractility.

The conventional perception is that inflammation in Crohn's disease is transmural, while that in ulcerative colitis is limited to the mucosa. This concept might have developed from morphological observations of significant infiltration of white blood cells in the muscle layers of Crohn's disease but not in those of ulcerative colitis. However, this concept is not consistent with the fact that inflammation in both types of IBD similarly suppresses circular muscle contractility [413, 434–436]. There is no known mechanism by which inflammation confined to the mucosa impairs smooth muscle function, since smooth muscle impairment in inflammation requires local release of inflammatory mediators in the muscularis externa.

Studies on the experimental models of Crohn's colitis and ulcerative colitis—trinitrobenzene sulfonic (TNBS) acid- and dextran sodium (DSS)-induced colonic inflammations, respectively [433, 444, 445]—show that the inflammatory mediators and their genetic targets to suppress circular smooth muscle contractility differ markedly between the two types of colonic inflammation.

Recent studies in animal models of the two forms of IBD and accumulating clinical findings [446, 447] suggest that inflammation is transmural in both forms of IBD. Crohn's colitis–like inflammation is due to transmural generation of oxidative stress and peptide inflammatory mediators. The ulcerative colitis–like inflammation is primarily due to transmural generation of oxidative stress. Peptide inflammatory mediators play a minor role in ulcerative colitis–like inflammation. Oxidative stress (H_2O_2) suppresses the $G\alpha_q$ protein of the excitation-contraction coupling in smooth muscle cells to suppress their contractility. By contrast, cytokines, such as IL-1β, suppress the α_{1C}-subunit and CPI-17 proteins of the excitation-contraction coupling to suppress circular smooth muscle reactivity to ACh [446].

Both types of inflammation begin with a breakdown of the mucosal barrier, exposing the sterile interior of the colon wall to a pathogenic luminal environment. The breakdown of the mucosal barrier by TNBS results in the translocation of luminal bacteria across the colon wall within 24 hours [448]. TNBS impairs the epithelial barrier function by necrosis. By contrast, Toll-like receptor 4 (TLR4) signaling, which limits bacterial translocation, mediates DSS inflammatory response [449, 450]. DSS arrests the epithelial cell cycle, resulting in apoptosis, impaired proliferation, and weak release of peptide inflammatory mediators [451–453]. DSS inflammation can occur in germ-free or severely-combined-immunodeficiency (SCID) mice [454, 455]. Consequently, bacterial translocation is marginal and confined to the mucosa, indicating its lesser role in DSS inflammation than in TNBS inflammation.

Taken together, aggressive bacterial translocation in TNBS inflammation may underlie the transmural infiltration of immune cells and release of cytokines/chemokines. On the other hand, limited bacterial translocation results in much smaller infiltration of immune cells and release of cytokines/chemokines in the mucosa/submucosa of DSS inflammation. It is noteworthy that TNBS inflammation in the absence of intestinal flora is also primarily mucosal [448]. The differences in the nature of the damage to the epithelium (e.g., apoptosis and necrosis) may underlie the two strikingly different types of inflammatory responses in TNBS and DSS.

Enteric Neuronal Dysfunction

Together with smooth muscle cells, the enteric neurons play an essential role in regulating motility function. They are in the same hostile inflammatory environment as the smooth muscle cells, but their precise role in impaired motility dysfunction in colonic inflammation remains ambiguous. This is largely due to the lack of availability of neuronal cultures until recently [456], the multiple types of neurons containing more than one neurotransmitter, and our limited ability to correlate neuronal abnormality with motor dysfunction. Immunohistochemical studies on inflamed and normal tissues have yielded mixed results [457–461].

Morphological data show that inflammation does not alter the density of neurons innervating circular smooth muscle cells [462]. However, it may impair the packaging, storage, and release of neurotransmitters from the nerve endings of motor and sympathetic neurons [463–465]. Impairment in the synthesis/release of ACh will suppress in vivo motor activity by reduced stimulation of excitation-contraction coupling in smooth muscle cells. Electrophysiological studies show that inflammation in guinea pig colon enhances the excitability of AH neurons and facilitates synaptic transmission in S neurons [466, 467]. However, we do not know yet how these changes relate to the suppression of neurotransmitter release, suppression of RPCs, and the stimulation of GMCs during inflammation.

The number of ICC-MP in the affected areas of Crohn's disease does not differ from that in controls, whereas the number of ICC-IM decreases and that of ICC-DMP increases [457]. However, recent publications have discounted any role of ICC in regulating motility function [79, 365, 468]. In spite of the changes found in the number of ICCs or damage to their processes, the slow waves and nitrergic inhibition seem to be normal in inflammation, as discussed above.

Take-home Messages

1. Impairment of excitation-contraction coupling in smooth muscle cells due to suppression of key cell-signaling proteins by inflammatory mediators contributes to the suppression of RPCs and tone in the colons of human IBD patients and in animal models of inflammation.
2. Inflammation impairs the release of neurotransmitters from enteric motor neurons.
3. We do not know the cellular mechanisms by which colonic inflammation enhances the frequency of GMCs.

Diverticular Disease

Diverticular disease is prevalent in up to 30% of the population over sixty years of age—about 15% of these patients go on to develop clinical symptoms [469–473]. Clinically, these patients are divided into three categories: asymptomatic diverticular disease, symptomatic uncomplicated diverticular disease, and symptomatic complicated diverticular disease. Some complications of diverticular disease—perforation, fistula, or bowel obstruction—relate to the severity and duration of colitis. The following discussion focuses primarily on asymptomatic and symptomatic diverticular disease patients.

The symptoms of diverticular disease include recurrent abdominal pain in the lower left quadrant and altered bowel habits: diarrhea, constipation, or alternating diarrhea (loose stools) and constipation (hard stools). Additional secondary symptoms are bloating, straining, urgency, incontinence, and mucus and blood in stools [404, 473–475]. These symptoms generally develop in patients over the age of 50 years. Low fiber in the diet is a likely contributor to its higher prevalence in Western counties. However, there is no hard evidence for it. The diverticula form primarily in the sigmoid colon. The severity of the symptoms relates to the degree of diverticulitis [476].

The symptoms of diverticulitis overlap with those of IBD and IBS-D, i.e., abdominal cramping accompanied by altered bowel habits. However, the etiologies of the two conditions may differ to some degree. In IBS-D, inflammation plays little role in the induction of these symptoms. A randomized double-blind placebo-controlled study found little improvement in IBS symptoms in IBS-PI patients by prednisone treatment [354]. We do not fully understand the events leading up to inflammation in IBD patients. However, in IBD, inflammation evenly covers the affected segment. Prednisone treatment is a major therapy in IBD patients. In diverticulitis, the inflammation starts by the translocation of pathogenic fecal material into the diverticula, causing abscess formation. Therefore, in diverticular disease, inflammation occurs in pockets centered on diverticula, and it may be unevenly distributed through the muscle layer. The circular muscle layer in diverticulitis shows hypertrophy and hyperplasia [473, 477, 478].

Colonic Motor Dysfunction in Diverticular Disease Patients

Manometric recordings show a higher incidence of GMCs in the sigmoid colon (and distal to it) in symptomatic diverticular disease patients than in asymptomatic patients or healthy controls. Overall motor activity, quantified as total duration of contractions, is also higher in symptomatic (complicated or uncomplicated) diverticular disease patients than in asymptomatic patients or in normal healthy subjects [476, 479, 480].

Take-home Messages

1. Although, diverticular disease involves inflammation in the diverticula, its symptoms in symptomatic patients are similar to those of IBS-D, i.e., abdominal cramping, diarrhea with loose stools, and alternating diarrhea and constipation.

2. Diarrhea with loose stools is a result of an increase in the frequency of GMCs.

Cellular and Molecular Mechanisms

Pioneering studies in diverticular disease patients proposed that the diverticula form by high outward pressures generated in the lumen [481, 482]. These studies did not identify the source of the pressure. Our current understanding of risk factors for the formation of diverticula are:

1. Strong compression of the colon wall by GMCs can generate high outward pressure.
2. A low-residue diet can create hard stools due to lack of fiber content [483–485].
3. Muscle tensile strength decreases with age [486–492].
4. The sigmoid colon wall near the entry of blood vessels is weaker than at other regions.

Based on these understandings, a potential sequence of events leading to diverticulitis is:

1. A low-fiber diet results in lesser retention of water in feces, causing them to harden.
2. Colonic GMCs occur spontaneously up to about 10 times a day in normal subjects. When a GMC strongly squeezes over a hardened stool pellet, it generates a bulge.
3. Weaker tensile strength of the colon wall increases the risk that the bulge will herniate the colon wall to form a diverticulum. Note that it might take repeated incidents to form a diverticulum.
4. Thereafter, colonic contractions, especially the GMCs, push the pathogenic fecal material into the diverticula.
5. The diverticula do not generate contractions to expel the fecal material.
6. The trapped fecal material starts infection, resulting in an inflammatory response and abscess formation.
7. The continuity of the muscle layers between the diverticula and the unaffected colon spreads inflammation to neighboring smooth muscle cells.
8. Inflammation in muscularis externa causes enteric neuronal and smooth muscle dysfunction to increase the frequency of GMCs as well as induce visceral hypersensitivity.
9. The inflammation that begins in the diverticula becomes transmural [473].

Note that the formation of diverticula by itself does not generate the symptoms of pain and altered bowel habits. The symptoms of intermittent abdominal cramping and altered bowel habits result primarily from the increase in the frequency of GMCs at the site of the inflamed diverticula. The GMCs that propagate to the rectum induce urgency and frequent defecation. As noted earlier [419, 421, 422], frequent GMCs rupture the mucosal barrier in the inflamed colon segment to cause bleeding and exudation of mucus, both expelled with the stool. The stool is loose because frequent mass movements by GMCs reduce its contact time with the mucosa in the sigmoid colon.

Diverticulitis patients show the same phenomena as IBD patients, sometimes passing loose stools, sometimes hard stools. Manometric data during the two conditions are not available. The frequency of GMCs likely fluctuates above and below normal levels to produce alternating diarrhea and constipation.

The amplitude of GMCs in diverticulitis—110 to 120 mmHg [476]—is about the same as that in normal subjects: 115 mmHg [28, 195, 197]. Therefore, pain in these patients is likely due to inflammation-induced visceral hypersensitivity to colorectal distension by a balloon or its compression by a GMC (see Figure 37C). The sigmoid colon bearing the diverticula and the rectum are hypersensitivity to luminal distension without a change in their compliance [493].

Diverticular disease patients tend to have raised scores on the Hospital Anxiety and Depression scale [494]. Whether a cause-and-effect relationship exists between an increase in anxiety/depression and colonic pain is unknown. However, it seems likely that these patients develop higher anxiety/depression scores following the development of frequent and debilitating colonic pain.

A recent animal study shows that bacterial translocation to the muscularis externa enhances the expression of insulin growth factor-1 (IGF-1) and transformation growth factor-β (TGF-β) in the muscularis externa, causing hypertrophy and hyperplasia, thus thickening the muscle layers [446]. No data are available on changes in the expressions of these growth factors in symptomatic diverticular disease patients. One may speculate, however, that similar changes might induce thickening of muscle layers in diverticular disease patients [477, 478].

Immunofluorescence findings show that inflammation in diverticular disease alters the expressions of several endogenous peptides, including substance P (SP), galanin, neuropeptides K (NPK), pituitary adenylate cyclase–activating peptide (PACAP), and vasoactive intestinal polypeptide (VIP). However, the cause-and-effect relationship between these changes and the symptoms of diverticular disease are unknown. Recent studies in human colonic smooth muscle cells show that VIP regulates transcription of the α_{1C}-subunit of $Ca_v1.2b$ (L-type) calcium channels in circular smooth muscle cells [173]. The influx of calcium, essential for smooth muscle contraction, occurs through these channels. Therefore, an increase in the expression of these channels enhances calcium influx, the amplitude of contractions, and colonic transit [174, 355]. The twofold increase of VIP in the circular muscle layer of the colon of symptomatic diverticular disease patients might be a contributing factor in the increased frequency of GMCs in diverticulitis.

. . . .

References

[1]   Cowles VE, Sarna SK. Relation between small intestinal motor activity and transit in secretory diarrhea. *Am J Physiol* 1990;259:G420–9.

[2]   Johnson CP, Sarna SK, Baytiyeh R, Zhu YR, Cowles VE, Telford GL, Roza AM, Adams MB. Postprandial motor activity and its relationship to transit in the canine ileum. *Surgery* 1997;121:182–9.

[3]   Sethi AK, Sarna SK. Contractile mechanisms of canine colonic propulsion. *Am J Physiol* 1995;268:G530–8.

[4]   Sarna SK. Colonic motor activity. *Surg Clin North Am* 1993;73:1201–23.

[5]   Haba T, Sarna SK. Regulation of gastroduodenal emptying of solids by gastropyloroduodenal contractions. *Am J Physiol* 1993;264:G261–71.

[6]   Sarna SK. Giant migrating contractions and their myoelectric correlates in the small intestine. *Am J Physiol* 1987;253:G697–705.

[7]   Lang IM, Sarna SK, Condon RE. Gastrointestinal motor correlates of vomiting in the dog: quantification and characterization as an independent phenomenon. *Gastroenterology* 1986;90:40–7.

[8]   Karaus M, Sarna SK. Giant migrating contractions during defecation in the dog colon. *Gastroenterology* 1987;92:925–33.

[9]   Otterson MF, Sarna SK. Neural control of small intestinal giant migrating contractions. *Am J Physiol* 1994;266:G576–84.

[10]   Bassotti G, Iantorno G, Fiorella S, Bustos-Fernandez L, Bilder CR. Colonic motility in man: features in normal subjects and in patients with chronic idiopathic constipation. *Am J Gastroenterol* 1999;94:1760–70.

[11]   Shi G, Ergun GA, Manka M, Kahrilas PJ. Lower esophageal sphincter relaxation characteristics using a sleeve sensor in clinical manometry. *Am J Gastroenterol* 1998;93:2373–9.

[12]   Li M, Johnson CP, Adams MB, Sarna SK. Cholinergic and nitrergic regulation of in vivo giant migrating contractions in rat colon. *Am J Physiol Gastrointest Liver Physiol* 2002;283: G544–52.

[13]   Fida R, Lyster DJ, Bywater RA, Taylor GS. Colonic migrating motor complexes (CMMCs) in the isolated mouse colon. *Neurogastroenterol Motil* 1997;9:99–107.

[14]   Bush TG, Spencer NJ, Watters N, Sanders KM, Smith TK. Spontaneous migrating motor complexes occur in both the terminal ileum and colon of the C57BL/6 mouse in vitro. *Auton Neurosci* 2000;84:162–8.

[15]   Gourcerol G, Wang L, Adelson DW, Larauche M, Tache Y, Million M. Cholinergic giant migrating contractions in conscious mouse colon assessed by using a novel noninvasive solid-state manometry method: modulation by stressors. *Am J Physiol Gastrointest Liver Physiol* 2009;296:G992–1002.

[16]   Gonzalez A, Sarna SK. Neural regulation of in vitro giant contractions in the rat colon. *Am J Physiol Gastrointest Liver Physiol* 2001;281:G275–82.

[17]   Gonzalez A, Sarna SK. Different types of contractions in rat colon and their modulation by oxidative stress. *Am J Physiol Gastrointest Liver Physiol* 2001;280:G546–54.

[18]   Hipper K, Ehrlein HJ. Motility of the large intestine and flow of digesta in pigs. *Res Vet Sci* 2001;71:93–100.

[19]   Coulie B, Camilleri M, Bharucha AE, Sandborn WJ, Burton D. Colonic motility in chronic ulcerative proctosigmoiditis and the effects of nicotine on colonic motility in patients and healthy subjects. *Aliment Pharmacol Ther* 2001;15:653–63.

[20]   Ford MJ, Camilleri M, Wiste JA, Hanson RB. Differences in colonic tone and phasic response to a meal in the transverse and sigmoid human colon. *Gut* 1995;37:264–9.

[21]   Coffin B, Lemann M, Flourie B, Picon L, Rambaud JC, Jian R. Ileal tone in humans: effects of locoregional distensions and eating. *Am J Physiol* 1994;267:G569–74.

[22]   Chey WY, Jin HO, Lee MH, Sun SW, Lee KY. Colonic motility abnormality in patients with irritable bowel syndrome exhibiting abdominal pain and diarrhea. *Am J Gastroenterol* 2001;96:1499–506.

[23]   Sarna SK. Enteric descending and afferent neural signaling stimulated by giant migrating contractions: essential contributing factors to visceral pain. *Am J Physiol Gastrointest Liver Physiol* 2007;292:G572–81.

[24]   Bayliss W, Starling E. The movements and innervation of small intestine. *J Physiol* 1899; 24:99–143.

[25]   Sarna SK, Soergel KH, Harig JM, Loo FD, Wood CM, Donahue KM, Ryan RP, Arndorfer RC. Spatial and temporal patterns of human jejunal contractions. *Am J Physiol* 1989;257: G423–32.

[26]   Johnson CP, Sarna SK, Cowles VE, Baytiyeh R, Zhu YR, Buchmann E, Bonham L, Roza AM, Adams MB. Effects of transection and reanastomosis on postprandial jejunal transit and contractile activity. *Surgery* 1995;117:531–7.

[27]   Quigley EM, Phillips SF, Dent J. Distinctive patterns of interdigestive motility at the ca-
       nine ileocolonic junction. *Gastroenterology* 1984;87:836–44.

[28]   Rao SS, Sadeghi P, Beaty J, Kavlock R, Ackerson K. Ambulatory 24-h colonic manometry
       in healthy humans. *Am J Physiol Gastrointest Liver Physiol* 2001;280:G629–39.

[29]   Sarna SK. Myoelectric correlates of colonic motor complexes and contractile activity. *Am J
       Physiol* 1986;250:G213–20.

[30]   Sarna S, Latimer P, Campbell D, Waterfall WE. Electrical and contractile activities of the
       human rectosigmoid. *Gut* 1982;23:698–705.

[31]   Bueno L, Fioramonti J, Ruckebusch Y, Frexinos J, Coulom P. Evaluation of colonic myo-
       electrical activity in health and functional disorders. *Gut* 1980;21:480–5.

[32]   Powell AK, Fida R, Bywater RA. Motility in the isolated mouse colon: migrating motor
       complexes, myoelectric complexes and pressure waves. *Neurogastroenterol Motil* 2003;15:
       257–66.

[33]   Bassotti G, Crowell MD, Cheskin LJ, Chami TN, Schuster MM, Whitehead WE. Physi-
       ological correlates of colonic motility in patients with irritable bowel syndrome. *Z Gastro-
       enterol* 1998;36:811–7.

[34]   Narducci F, Bassotti G, Gaburri M, Morelli A. Twenty four hour manometric recording of
       colonic motor activity in healthy man. *Gut* 1987;28:17–25.

[35]   Matsushima Y. [Studies on colonic motor correlates of spontaneous defecation in conscious
       dogs]. *Nippon Heikatsukin Gakkai Zasshi* 1989;25:137–46.

[36]   Bampton PA, Dinning PG, Kennedy ML, Lubowski DZ, deCarle D, Cook IJ. Spatial and
       temporal organization of pressure patterns throughout the unprepared colon during spon-
       taneous defecation. *Am J Gastroenterol* 2000;95:1027–35.

[37]   Lemann M, Flourie B, Picon L, Coffin B, Jian R, Rambaud JC. Motor activity recorded in
       the unprepared colon of healthy humans. *Gut* 1995;37:649–53.

[38]   Cook IJ, Furukawa Y, Panagopoulos V, Collins PJ, Dent J. Relationships between spatial
       patterns of colonic pressure and individual movements of content. *Am J Physiol Gastrointest
       Liver Physiol* 2000;278:G329–41.

[39]   Bassotti G, de Roberto G, Chistolini F, Sietchiping-Nzepa F, Morelli O, Morelli A.
       Twenty-four-hour manometric study of colonic propulsive activity in patients with diarrhea
       due to inflammatory (ulcerative colitis) and non-inflammatory (irritable bowel syndrome)
       conditions. *Int J Colorectal Dis* 2004;19:493–7.

[40]   Clemens CH, Samsom M, Van Berge Henegouwen GP, Smout AJ. Abnormalities of left
       colonic motility in ambulant nonconstipated patients with irritable bowel syndrome. *Dig Dis
       Sci* 2003;48:74–82.

[41]   Furness J. *The Enteric Nervous System.* Blackwell, 2006.

[42]   Narducci F, Bassotti G, Daniotti S, Del Soldato P, Pelli MA, Morelli A. Identification of muscarinic receptor subtype mediating colonic response to eating. *Dig Dis Sci* 1985;30: 124–8.

[43]   Narducci F, Bassotti G, Granata MT, Pelli MA, Gaburri M, Palumbo R, Morelli A. Colonic motility and gastric emptying in patients with irritable bowel syndrome. Effect of pretreatment with octylonium bromide. *Dig Dis Sci* 1986;31:241–6.

[44]   Sullivan MA, Cohen S, Snape WJ, Jr. Colonic myoelectrical activity in irritable-bowel syndrome. Effect of eating and anticholinergics. *N Engl J Med* 1978;298:878–83.

[45]   Sarna SK, Gonzalez A, Ryan RP. Enteric locus of action of prokinetics: ABT-229, motilin, and erythromycin. *Am J Physiol Gastrointest Liver Physiol* 2000;278:G744–52.

[46]   Costa M, Cuello AC, Furness JB, Franco R. Distribution of enteric neurons showing immunoreactivity for substance P in the guinea-pig ileum. *Neuroscience* 1980;5:323–31.

[47]   Grider JR. Identification of neurotransmitters regulating intestinal peristaltic reflex in humans. *Gastroenterology* 1989;97:1414–9.

[48]   Grider JR. Tachykinins as transmitters of ascending contractile component of the peristaltic reflex. *Am J Physiol* 1989;257:G709–14.

[49]   Furness JB. Types of neurons in the enteric nervous system. *J Auton Nerv Syst* 2000;81: 87–96.

[50]   Grider JR. Interplay of VIP and nitric oxide in regulation of the descending relaxation phase of peristalsis. *Am J Physiol* 1993;264:G334–40.

[51]   Grider JR, Jin JG. Distinct populations of sensory neurons mediate the peristaltic reflex elicited by muscle stretch and mucosal stimulation. *J Neurosci* 1994;14:2854–60.

[52]   Murthy KS. Signaling for contraction and relaxation in smooth muscle of the gut. *Annu Rev Physiol* 2006;68:345–74.

[53]   Somlyo AP, Somlyo AV. Ca2+ sensitivity of smooth muscle and nonmuscle myosin II: modulated by G proteins, kinases, and myosin phosphatase. *Physiol Rev* 2003;83:1325–58.

[54]   Brozovich FV. Myosin light chain phosphatase: it gets around. Circ Res 2002;90:500–2.

[55]   Hartshorne DJ, Ito M, Erdodi F. Myosin light chain phosphatase: subunit composition, interactions and regulation. *J Muscle Res Cell Motil* 1998;19:325–41.

[56]   Somlyo AP, Somlyo AV. Signal transduction by G-proteins, rho-kinase and protein phosphatase to smooth muscle and non-muscle myosin II. *J Physiol* 2000;522(Pt 2):177–85.

[57]   Lu G, Qian X, Berezin I, Telford GL, Huizinga JD, Sarna SK. Inflammation modulates in vitro colonic myoelectric and contractile activity and interstitial cells of Cajal. *Am J Physiol* 1997;273:G1233–45.

[58]   Rich A, Kenyon JL, Hume JR, Overturf K, Horowitz B, Sanders KM. Dihydropyridine-sensitive calcium channels expressed in canine colonic smooth muscle cells. *Am J Physiol* 1993;264:C745–54.

[59]   Huizinga JD, Stern HS, Chow E, Diamant NE, el-Sharkawy TY. Electrical basis of excitation and inhibition of human colonic smooth muscle. *Gastroenterology* 1986;90:1197–204.

[60]   Serio R, Barajas-Lopez C, Daniel EE, Berezin I, Huizinga JD. Slow-wave activity in colon: role of network of submucosal interstitial cells of Cajal. *Am J Physiol* 1991;260:G636–45.

[61]   Sato K, Sanders KM, Gerthoffer WT, Publicover NG. Sources of calcium utilized in cholinergic responses in canine colonic smooth muscle. *Am J Physiol* 1994;267:C1666–73.

[62]   Liu X, Rusch NJ, Striessnig J, Sarna SK. Down-regulation of L-type calcium channels in inflamed circular smooth muscle cells of the canine colon. *Gastroenterology* 2001;120: 480–9.

[63]   Liu XR, Rusch NJ, Striessnig J, Sarna SK. Down-regulation of L-type calcium channels in inflamed circular smooth muscle cells of the canine colon. *Gastroenterology* 2001;120: 480–489.

[64]   Huizinga JD, Waterfall WE. Electrical correlate of circumferential contractions in human colonic circular muscle. *Gut* 1988;29:10–6.

[65]   Sanders KM. Excitation-contraction coupling without Ca2+ action potentials in small intestine. *Am J Physiol* 1983;244:C356–61.

[66]   Large WA. Receptor-operated Ca2(+)-permeable nonselective cation channels in vascular smooth muscle: a physiologic perspective. *J Cardiovasc Electrophysiol* 2002;13:493–501.

[67]   Ji G, Barsotti RJ, Feldman ME, Kotlikoff MI. Stretch-induced calcium release in smooth muscle. *J Gen Physiol* 2002;119:533–44.

[68]   Kirber MT, Walsh JV, Jr., Singer JJ. Stretch-activated ion channels in smooth muscle: a mechanism for the initiation of stretch-induced contraction. *Pflugers Arch* 1988;412:339–45.

[69]   Felder CC. Muscarinic acetylcholine receptors: signal transduction through multiple effectors. *Faseb J* 1995;9:619–25.

[70]   Eglen RM, Reddy H, Watson N, Challiss RA. Muscarinic acetylcholine receptor subtypes in smooth muscle. *Trends Pharmacol Sci* 1994;15:114–9.

[71]   Wess J, Liu J, Blin N, Yun J, Lerche C, Kostenis E. Structural basis of receptor/G protein coupling selectivity studied with muscarinic receptors as model systems. *Life Sci* 1997; 60:1007–14.

[72]   McFadzean I, Gibson A. The developing relationship between receptor-operated and store-operated calcium channels in smooth muscle. *Br J Pharmacol* 2002;135:1–13.

[73]   Sarna SK, Bardakjian BL, Waterfall WE, Lind JF. Human colonic electrical control activity (ECA). *Gastroenterology* 1980;78:1526–36.

[74]   Snape WJ, Jr., Carlson GM, Cohen S. Colonic myoelectric activity in the irritable bowel syndrome. *Gastroenterology* 1976;70:326–30.

[75]   Taylor I, Duthie HL, Smallwood R, Linkens D. Large bowel myoelectrical activity in man. *Gut* 1975;16:808–14.

[76]   Provenzale L, Pisano M. Methods for recording electrical activity of the human colon in vivo. Clinical applications. *Am J Dig Dis* 1971;16:712–22.

[77]   Couturier D, Roze C, Couturier-Turpin MH, Debray C. Electromyography of the colon in situ. An experimental study in man and in the rabbit. *Gastroenterology* 1969;56:317–22.

[78]   Sanders KM, Koh SD, Ward SM. Interstitial cells of Cajal as pacemakers in the gastrointestinal tract. *Annu Rev Physiol* 2006;68:307–43.

[79]   Sarna SK. Are interstitial cells of Cajal plurifunction cells in the gut? *Am J Physiol Gastrointest Liver Physiol* 2008;294:G372–90.

[80]   Murthy KS. cAMP inhibits IP(3)-dependent Ca(2+) release by preferential activation of cGMP-primed PKG. *Am J Physiol Gastrointest Liver Physiol* 2001;281:G1238–45.

[81]   Huber A, Trudrung P, Storr M, Franck H, Schusdziarra V, Ruth P, Allescher HD. Protein kinase G expression in the small intestine and functional importance for smooth muscle relaxation. *Am J Physiol* 1998;275:G629–37.

[82]   Jiang H, Colbran JL, Francis SH, Corbin JD. Direct evidence for cross-activation of cGMP-dependent protein kinase by cAMP in pig coronary arteries. *J Biol Chem* 1992;267:1015–9.

[83]   Jin JG, Murthy KS, Grider JR, Makhlouf GM. Activation of distinct cAMP- and cGMP-dependent pathways by relaxant agents in isolated gastric muscle cells. *Am J Physiol* 1993;264:G470–7.

[84]   Murthy KS, Zhou H, Grider JR, Makhlouf GM. Inhibition of sustained smooth muscle contraction by PKA and PKG preferentially mediated by phosphorylation of RhoA. *Am J Physiol Gastrointest Liver Physiol* 2003;284:G1006–16.

[85]   Daniel EaS, SK. The generation and conduction of activitry in smooth muscle, 1978.

[86]   Nelsen TS, Becker JC. Simulation of the electrical and mechanical gradient of the small intestine. *Am J Physiol* 1968;214:749–57.

[87]   Sarna SK, Daniel EE, Kingma YJ. Simulation of slow-wave electrical activity of small intestine. *Am J Physiol* 1971;221:166–75.

[88]   Sarna SK, Daniel EE, Kingma YJ. Simulation of the electric-control activity of the stomach by an array of relaxation oscillators. *Am J Dig Dis* 1972;17:299–310.

[89]   Diamant NE, Bortoff A. Nature of the intestinal low-wave frequency gradient. *Am J Physiol* 1969;216:301–7.

[90]   Smith TK, Reed JB, Sanders KM. Origin and propagation of electrical slow waves in circular muscle of canine proximal colon. *Am J Physiol* 1987;252:C215–24.

[91]   Smith TK, Reed JB, Sanders KM. Effects of membrane potential on electrical slow waves of canine proximal colon. *Am J Physiol* 1988;255:C828–34.

[92]   Bauer AJ, Sanders KM. Gradient in excitation-contraction coupling in canine gastric antral circular muscle. *J Physiol* 1985;369:283–94.

[93] Horiguchi K, Semple GS, Sanders KM, Ward SM. Distribution of pacemaker function through the tunica muscularis of the canine gastric antrum. *J Physiol* 2001;537:237–50.

[94] Malysz J, Thuneberg L, Mikkelsen HB, Huizinga JD. Action potential generation in the small intestine of W mutant mice that lack interstitial cells of Cajal. *Am J Physiol* 1996;271: G387–99.

[95] Szurszewski JH, Farrugia G. Carbon monoxide is an endogenous hyperpolarizing factor in the gastrointestinal tract. *Neurogastroenterol Motil* 2004;16 Suppl 1:81–5.

[96] Hagger R, Gharaie S, Finlayson C, Kumar D. Regional and transmural density of interstitial cells of Cajal in human colon and rectum. *Am J Physiol* 1998;275:G1309–16.

[97] Rumessen JJ, Peters S, Thuneberg L. Light- and electron microscopical studies of interstitial cells of Cajal and muscle cells at the submucosal border of human colon. *Lab Invest* 1993;68:481–95.

[98] Faussone-Pellegrini MS, Pantalone D, Cortesini C. Smooth muscle cells, interstitial cells of Cajal and myenteric plexus interrelationships in the human colon. *Acta Anat (Basel)* 1990; 139:31–44.

[99] He CL, Burgart L, Wang L, Pemberton J, Young-Fadok T, Szurszewski J, Farrugia G. Decreased interstitial cell of cajal volume in patients with slow-transit constipation. *Gastroenterology* 2000;118:14–21.

[100] Alberti E, Mikkelsen HB, Wang X, Diaz M, Larsen JO, Huizinga JD, Jimenez M. Pacemaker activity and inhibitory neurotransmission in the colon of Ws/Ws mutant rats. *Am J Physiol Gastrointest Liver Physiol* 2007.

[101] Sanders KM, Publicover NG, Ward SM. Involvement of interstitial cells of Cajal in pacemaker activity of canine colon. *J Smooth Muscle Res* 1991;27:1–11.

[102] Farrugia G, Lei S, Lin X, Miller SM, Nath KA, Ferris CD, Levitt M, Szurszewski JH. A major role for carbon monoxide as an endogenous hyperpolarizing factor in the gastrointestinal tract. *Proc Natl Acad Sci USA* 2003;100:8567–70.

[103] Wood JD. Physiology of the enteric nervous system. Raven, 1994.

[104] Lomax AE, Furness JB. Neurochemical classification of enteric neurons in the guinea-pig distal colon. *Cell Tissue Res* 2000;302:59–72.

[105] Costa M, Brookes SJ, Steele PA, Gibbins I, Burcher E, Kandiah CJ. Neurochemical classification of myenteric neurons in the guinea-pig ileum. *Neuroscience* 1996;75:949–67.

[106] Timmermans JP, Adriaensen D, Cornelissen W, Scheuermann DW. Structural organization and neuropeptide distribution in the mammalian enteric nervous system, with special attention to those components involved in mucosal reflexes. *Comp Biochem Physiol A Physiol* 1997;118:331–40.

[106a] Gershon MD, Tack J. The serotonin signaling system: from basic understanding to drug development for functional GI disorders. *Gastroenterology* 2007;132(1): p. 397–414.

[107] Dogiel A. Uber den Bau der Ganglien in den Geflechten des Darmes und der Gallenblase des Menschen und der Saugetiere. *Arch Anat Physiol Leipzig Anat Abt Jg* 1899:130–158.

[108] Cornelissen W, de Laet A, Kroese AB, van Bogaert PP, Scheuermann DW, Timmermans JP. Excitatory synaptic inputs on myenteric Dogiel type II neurones of the pig ileum. *J Comp Neurol* 2001;432:137–54.

[109] Palmer JM, Schemann M, Tamura K, Wood JD. Calcitonin gene-related peptide excites myenteric neurons. *Eur J Pharmacol* 1986;132:163–70.

[110] Lomax AE, Sharkey KA, Bertrand PP, Low AM, Bornstein JC, Furness JB. Correlation of morphology, electrophysiology and chemistry of neurons in the myenteric plexus of the guinea-pig distal colon. *J Auton Nerv Syst* 1999;76:45–61.

[111] Nurgali K, Stebbing MJ, Furness JB. Correlation of electrophysiological and morphological characteristics of enteric neurons in the mouse colon. *J Comp Neurol* 2004;468:112–24.

[112] Takahashi A, Tomomasa T, Kaneko H, Hatori R, Ishige T, Suzuki M, Mochiki E, Morikawa A, Kuwano H. In vivo recording of colonic motility in conscious rats with deficiency of interstitial cells of Cajal, with special reference to the effects of nitric oxide on colonic motility. *J Gastroenterol* 2005;40:1043–8.

[113] Orihata M, Sarna SK. Inhibition of nitric oxide synthase delays gastric emptying of solid meals. *J Pharmacol Exp Ther* 1994;271:660–70.

[113a] Sarna SK et al.,Nitric oxide regulates migrating motor complex cycling and its postprandial disruption. *Am J Physiol* 1993;265(4 Pt 1):G749–66.

[114] Grider JR. Neurotransmitters mediating the intestinal peristaltic reflex in the mouse. *J Pharmacol Exp Ther* 2003;307:460–7.

[115] Grider JR, Makhlouf GM. Colonic peristaltic reflex: identification of vasoactive intestinal peptide as mediator of descending relaxation. *Am J Physiol* 1986;251:G40–5.

[116] Sarna SK. Neuronal locus and cellular signaling for stimulation of ileal giant migrating and phasic contractions. *Am J Physiol Gastrointest Liver Physiol* 2003;284:G789–97.

[117] Porter AJ, Wattchow DA, Brookes SJ, Costa M. The neurochemical coding and projections of circular muscle motor neurons in the human colon. *Gastroenterology* 1997;113:1916–23.

[118] Beckett EA, Takeda Y, Yanase H, Sanders KM, Ward SM. Synaptic specializations exist between enteric motor nerves and interstitial cells of Cajal in the murine stomach. *J Comp Neurol* 2005;493:193–206.

[119] Horiguchi K, Sanders KM, Ward SM. Enteric motor neurons form synaptic-like junctions with interstitial cells of Cajal in the canine gastric antrum. *Cell Tissue Res* 2003;311: 299–313.

[120] Wang XY, Paterson C, Huizinga JD. Cholinergic and nitrergic innervation of ICC-DMP and ICC-IM in the human small intestine. *Neurogastroenterol Motil* 2003;15:531–43.

[121] Faussone-Pellegrini MS, Pantalone D, Cortesini C. An ultrastructural study of the smooth muscle cells and nerve endings of the human stomach. *J Submicrosc Cytol Pathol* 1989;21: 421–37.

[122] Burns AJ, Lomax AE, Torihashi S, Sanders KM, Ward SM. Interstitial cells of Cajal mediate inhibitory neurotransmission in the stomach. *Proc Natl Acad Sci USA* 1996;93: 12008–13.

[123] Ward SM, Beckett EA, Wang X, Baker F, Khoyi M, Sanders KM. Interstitial cells of Cajal mediate cholinergic neurotransmission from enteric motor neurons. *J Neurosci* 2000; 20:1393–403.

[124] Altdorfer K, Bagameri G, Donath T, Feher E. Nitric oxide synthase immunoreactivity of interstitial cells of Cajal in experimental colitis. *Inflamm Res* 2002;51:569–71.

[125] Ward SM, Sanders KM. Interstitial cells of Cajal: primary targets of enteric motor innervation. *Anat Rec* 2001;262:125–35.

[126] Vannucchi MG, Corsani L, Bani D, Faussone-Pellegrini MS. Myenteric neurons and interstitial cells of Cajal of mouse colon express several nitric oxide synthase isoforms. *Neurosci Lett* 2002;326:191–5.

[127] Goyal RK, Chaudhury A. Mounting evidence against the role of ICC in neurotransmission to smooth muscle in the gut. *Am J Physiol Gastrointest Liver Physiol* 2009.

[128] Zhang Y, Carmichael SA, Wang XY, Huizinga JD, Paterson WG. Neurotransmission in lower esophageal Sphincter of W/Wv mutant mice. *Am J Physiol Gastrointest Liver Physiol* 2009.

[129] Herkenham M. Extrasynaptic receptors and parasynaptic communication in the brain. *Brain Res Bull* 1999;50:351–2.

[130] Nicholson C. Signals that go with the flow. *Trends Neurosci* 1999;22:143–5.

[131] Sykova E. Extrasynaptic volume transmission and diffusion parameters of the extracellular space. *Neuroscience* 2004;129:861–76.

[132] Vizi ES, Kiss JP, Lendvai B. Nonsynaptic communication in the central nervous system. *Neurochem Int* 2004;45:443–51.

[133] Porter AJ, Wattchow DA, Brookes SJ, Costa M. Cholinergic and nitrergic interneurones in the myenteric plexus of the human colon. *Gut* 2002;51:70–5.

[134] Frantzides CT, Sarna SK, Matsumoto T, Lang IM, Condon RE. An intrinsic neural pathway for long intestino-intestinal inhibitory reflexes. *Gastroenterology* 1987;92:594–603.

[135] Sarna S, Stoddard C, Belbeck L, McWade D. Intrinsic nervous control of migrating myoelectric complexes. *Am J Physiol* 1981;241:G16–23.

[136] Wattchow DA, Porter AJ, Brookes SJ, Costa M. The polarity of neurochemically defined myenteric neurons in the human colon. *Gastroenterology* 1997;113:497–506.

[137] Nichols K, Staines W, Krantis A. Neural sites of the human colon colocalize nitric oxide synthase-related NADPH diaphorase activity and neuropeptide Y. *Gastroenterology* 1994; 107:968–75.

[138] Burleigh DE, Furness JB. Distribution and actions of galanin and vasoactive intestinal peptide in the human colon. *Neuropeptides* 1990;16:77–82.

[139] Wardell CF, Bornstein JC, Furness JB. Projections of 5-hydroxytryptamine-immunoreactive neurons in guinea-pig distal colon. *Cell Tissue Res* 1994;278:379–87.

[140] Neunlist M, Dobreva G, Schemann M. Characteristics of mucosally projecting myenteric neurones in the guinea-pig proximal colon. *J Physiol* 1999;517(Pt 2):533–46.

[141] Kunze WA, Furness JB. The enteric nervous system and regulation of intestinal motility. *Annu Rev Physiol* 1999;61:117–42.

[142] Pan H, Gershon MD. Activation of intrinsic afferent pathways in submucosal ganglia of the guinea pig small intestine. *J Neurosci* 2000;20:3295–309.

[143] Wood JD. Enteric nervous system: reflexes, pattern generators and motility. *Curr Opin Gastroenterol* 2008;24:149–58.

[144] Wade PR, Wood JD. Electrical behavior of myenteric neurons in guinea pig distal colon. *Am J Physiol* 1988;254:G522–30.

[145] Messenger JP, Bornstein JC, Furness JB. Electrophysiological and morphological classification of myenteric neurons in the proximal colon of the guinea-pig. *Neuroscience* 1994;60: 227–44.

[146] Nurgali K, Furness JB, Stebbing MJ. Correlation of electrophysiology, shape and synaptic properties of myenteric AH neurons of the guinea pig distal colon. *Auton Neurosci* 2003; 103:50–64.

[147] Wade PR, Wood JD. Synaptic behavior of myenteric neurons in guinea pig distal colon. *Am J Physiol* 1988;255:G184–90.

[148] Brookes SJ, Ewart WR, Wingate DL. Intracellular recordings from myenteric neurones in the human colon. *J Physiol* 1987;390:305–18.

[149] Sarna SK. Effect of fluid perfusion and cleansing on canine colonic motor activity. *Am J Physiol* 1992;262:G62–8.

[150] Morse D, Sassone-Corsi P. Time after time: inputs to and outputs from the mammalian circadian oscillators. *Trends Neurosci* 2002;25:632–7.

[151] Stankiewicz M, Grolleau F, Kielbasiewicz E, Panek I, Lapied B, Pelhate M. [Spontaneous activity of neural membranes]. *Postepy Hig Med Dosw* 2002;56:255–62.

[152] Fricker D, Miles R. Interneurons, spike timing, and perception. *Neuron* 2001;32:771–4.

[153] Sarna SK. Cyclic motor activity; migrating motor complex: 1985. *Gastroenterology* 1985; 89:894–913.

[154] Frexinos J, Bueno L, Fioramonti J. Diurnal changes in myoelectric spiking activity of the human colon. *Gastroenterology* 1985;88:1104–10.

[155] Liu LW, Huizinga JD. Canine colonic circular muscle generates action potentials without the pacemaker component. *Can J Physiol Pharmacol* 1994;72:70–81.

[156] Gershon MD, Tack J. The serotonin signaling system: from basic understanding to drug development for functional GI disorders. *Gastroenterology* 2007;132:397–414.

[157] Graf S, Sarna SK. 5-HT-induced jejunal motor activity: enteric locus of action and receptor subtypes. *Am J Physiol* 1996;270:G992–1000.

[158] Schang JC, Hemond M, Hebert M, Pilote M. Myoelectrical activity and intraluminal flow in human sigmoid colon. *Dig Dis Sci* 1986;31:1331–7.

[159] Schang JC, Dapoigny M, Devroede G. Stimulation of colonic peristalsis by vasopressin: electromyographic study in normal subjects and patients with chronic idiopathic constipation. *Can J Physiol Pharmacol* 1987;65:2137–41.

[160] Pluja L, Alberti E, Fernandez E, Mikkelsen HB, Thuneberg L, Jimenez M. Evidence supporting presence of two pacemakers in rat colon. *Am J Physiol Gastrointest Liver Physiol* 2001; 281:G255–66.

[161] Lee CW, Sarna SK, Singaram C, Casper MA. Ca2+ channel blockade by verapamil inhibits GMCs and diarrhea during small intestinal inflammation. *Am J Physiol* 1997;273:G785–94.

[162] Biancani P, Harnett KM, Sohn UD, Rhim BY, Behar J, Hillemeier C, Bitar KN. Differential signal transduction pathways in cat lower esophageal sphincter tone and response to ACh. *Am J Physiol* 1994;266:G767–74.

[163] Tsukamoto M, Sarna SK, Condon RE. A novel motility effect of tachykinins in normal and inflamed colon. *Am J Physiol* 1997;272:G1607–14.

[164] Hou JY, Otterson MF, Sarna SK. Local effect of substance P on colonic motor activity in different experimental states. *Am J Physiol* 1989;256:G997–1004.

[165] Sethi AK, Sarna SK. Colonic motor response to a meal in acute colitis. *Gastroenterology* 1991;101:1537–46.

[166] Sethi AK, Sarna SK. Colonic motor activity in acute colitis in conscious dogs. *Gastroenterology* 1991;100:954–63.

[167] Sarna SK. Differential signal transduction pathways to stimulate colonic giant migrating and phasic contractions. *Gastroenterology* 2000;118:A837.

[168] Olofsson B. Rho guanine dissociation inhibitors: pivotal molecules in cellular signalling. *Cell Signal* 1999;11:545–54.

[169] Fujihara H, Walker LA, Gong MC, Lemichez E, Boquet P, Somlyo AV, Somlyo AP. Inhibition of RhoA translocation and calcium sensitization by in vivo ADP-ribosylation with the chimeric toxin DC3B. *Mol Biol Cell* 1997;8:2437–47.

[170] Gong MC, Fujihara H, Somlyo AV, Somlyo AP. Translocation of rhoA associated with Ca2+ sensitization of smooth muscle. *J Biol Chem* 1997;272:10704–9.

[171] Murthy KS, Zhou H, Grider JR, Brautigan DL, Eto M, Makhlouf GM. Differential signalling by muscarinic receptors in smooth muscle: m2-mediated inactivation of myosin light chain kinase via Gi3, Cdc42/Rac1 and p21-activated kinase 1 pathway, and m3-mediated MLC20 (20 kDa regulatory light chain of myosin II) phosphorylation via Rho-associated kinase/myosin phosphatase targeting subunit 1 and protein kinase C/CPI-17 pathway. *Biochem J* 2003;374:145–55.

[172] Murthy KS, Grider JR, Kuemmerle JF, Makhlouf GM. Sustained muscle contraction induced by agonists, growth factors, and Ca(2+) mediated by distinct PKC isozymes. *Am J Physiol Gastrointest Liver Physiol* 2000;279:G201–10.

[173] Shi XZ, Choudhury BK, Pasricha PJ, Sarna SK. A novel role of VIP in colonic motility function: induction of excitation-transcription coupling in smooth muscle cells. *Gastroenterology* 2007;132:1388–400.

[174] Shi XZ, Sarna SK. Gene therapy of Cav1.2 channel with VIP and VIP receptor agonists and antagonists: a novel approach to designing promotility and antimotility agents. *Am J Physiol Gastrointest Liver Physiol* 2008;295:G187–G196.

[175] Lomax AE, Fernandez E, Sharkey KA. Plasticity of the enteric nervous system during intestinal inflammation. *Neurogastroenterol Motil* 2005;17:4–15.

[176] Shi XZ, Sarna SK. G protein-mediated dysfunction of excitation-contraction coupling in ileal inflammation. *Am J Physiol Gastrointest Liver Physiol* 2004;286:G899–905.

[177] Shi XZ, Sarna SK. Impairment of Ca(2+) mobilization in circular muscle cells of the inflamed colon. *Am J Physiol Gastrointest Liver Physiol* 2000;278:G234–42.

[178] Alvarez W. *An Introduction to Gastroenterology*. Paul B. Hoeber, 1948.

[179] Alvarez WCSE. Conduction in the small intestine. *Am J Physiol* 1919;26:99–143.

[180] White H, Rainey, WR, Monaghan, B and Harris, AS. Observations on the nervous control of the ileocecal sphincter and on intestinal movements in an unanesthetized human subject. *Am J Physiol* 1934;108:449–457.

[181] Roden S. An experimental study on intestinal movements; particularly with regard to ileus conditions in cases of trauma and peritonitis. *Acta Chirur Scandinavica* 1937;80:1–146.

[182] Kadowaki M, Wade PR, Gershon MD. Participation of 5-HT3, 5-HT4, and nicotinic receptors in the peristaltic reflex of guinea pig distal colon. *Am J Physiol* 1996;271:G849–57.

[183] Grider JR. Gastrin-releasing peptide is a modulatory neurotransmitter of the descending phase of the peristaltic reflex. *Am J Physiol Gastrointest Liver Physiol* 2004;287:G1109–15.

[184] Grider JR, Kuemmerle JF, Jin JG. 5-HT released by mucosal stimuli initiates peristalsis by

activating 5-HT4/5-HT1p receptors on sensory CGRP neurons. *Am J Physiol* 1996;270: G778–82.

[185] Costa M, Furness JB. The peristaltic reflex: an analysis of the nerve pathways and their pharmacology. *Naunyn Schmiedebergs Arch Pharmacol* 1976;294:47–60.

[186] Bian XC, Heffer LF, Gwynne RM, Bornstein JC, Bertrand PP. Synaptic transmission in simple motility reflex pathways excited by distension in guinea pig distal colon. *Am J Physiol Gastrointest Liver Physiol* 2004;287:G1017–27.

[187] Wade PR, Wood JD. Actions of serotonin and substance P on myenteric neurons of guinea-pig distal colon. *Eur J Pharmacol* 1988;148:1–8.

[188] Gershon MD. Review article: serotonin receptors and transporters—roles in normal and abnormal gastrointestinal motility. *Aliment Pharmacol Ther* 2004;20 Suppl 7:3–14.

[189] Latimer P, Sarna S, Campbell D, Latimer M, Waterfall W, Daniel EE. Colonic motor and myoelectrical activity: a comparative study of normal subjects, psychoneurotic patients, and patients with irritable bowel syndrome. *Gastroenterology* 1981;80:893–901.

[190] Kuriyama H, Osa T, Toida N. Nervous factors influencing the membrane activity of intestinal smooth muscle. *J Physiol* 1967;191:257–70.

[191] Kuriyama H, Osa T, Toida N. Electrophysiological study of the intestinal smooth muscle of the guinea-pig. *J Physiol* 1967;191:239–55.

[192] Donnelly G, Jackson TD, Ambrous K, Ye J, Safdar A, Farraway L, Huizinga JD. The myogenic component in distention-induced peristalsis in the guinea pig small intestine. *Am J Physiol Gastrointest Liver Physiol* 2001;280:G491–500.

[193] Jin JG, Foxx-Orenstein AE, Grider JR. Propulsion in guinea pig colon induced by 5-hydroxytryptamine (HT) via 5-HT4 and 5-HT3 receptors. *J Pharmacol Exp Ther* 1999; 288:93–7.

[194] Scott SM. Manometric techniques for the evaluation of colonic motor activity: current status. *Neurogastroenterol Motil* 2003;15:483–513.

[195] Bampton PA, Dinning PG, Kennedy ML, Lubowski DZ, Cook IJ. Prolonged multi-point recording of colonic manometry in the unprepared human colon: providing insight into potentially relevant pressure wave parameters. *Am J Gastroenterol* 2001;96:1838–48.

[196] Sloots CE, Felt-Bersma RJ. Effect of bowel cleansing on colonic transit in constipation due to slow transit or evacuation disorder. *Neurogastroenterol Motil* 2002;14:55–61.

[197] Bassotti G, Gaburri M. Manometric investigation of high-amplitude propagated contractile activity of the human colon. *Am J Physiol* 1988;255:G660–4.

[198] Hammer J, Phillips SF. Fluid loading of the human colon: effects on segmental transit and stool composition. *Gastroenterology* 1993;105:988–98.

[199] Proano M, Camilleri M, Phillips SF, Brown ML, Thomforde GM. Transit of solids through the human colon: regional quantification in the unprepared bowel. *Am J Physiol* 1990;258: G856–62.

[200] Furukawa Y, Cook IJ, Panagopoulos V, McEvoy RD, Sharp DJ, Simula M. Relationship between sleep patterns and human colonic motor patterns. *Gastroenterology* 1994;107:1372–81.

[201] Herbst F, Kamm MA, Morris GP, Britton K, Woloszko J, Nicholls RJ. Gastrointestinal transit and prolonged ambulatory colonic motility in health and faecal incontinence. *Gut* 1997;41:381–9.

[202] Soffer EE, Scalabrini P, Wingate DL. Prolonged ambulant monitoring of human colonic motility. *Am J Physiol* 1989;257:G601–6.

[203] Bassotti G, Gaburri M, Imbimbo BP, Rossi L, Farroni F, Pelli MA, Morelli A. Colonic mass movements in idiopathic chronic constipation. *Gut* 1988;29:1173–9.

[204] Kumar D, Wingate D, Ruckebusch Y. Circadian variation in the propagation velocity of the migrating motor complex. *Gastroenterology* 1986;91:926–30.

[205] Snyder F, Hobson JA, Morrison DF, Goldfrank F. Changes in respiration, heart rate, and systolic blood pressure in human sleep. *J Appl Physiol* 1964;19:417–22.

[206] Orem J. Medullary respiratory neuron activity: relationship to tonic and phasic REM sleep. *J Appl Physiol* 1980;48:54–65.

[207] Kline LR, Hendricks JC, Davies RO, Pack AI. Control of activity of the diaphragm in rapid-eye-movement sleep. *J Appl Physiol* 1986;61:1293–300.

[208] Niederau C, Faber S, Karaus M. Cholecystokinin's role in regulation of colonic motility in health and in irritable bowel syndrome. *Gastroenterology* 1992;102:1889–98.

[209] Snape WJ, Jr., Matarazzo SA, Cohen S. Effect of eating and gastrointestinal hormones on human colonic myoelectrical and motor activity. *Gastroenterology* 1978;75:373–8.

[210] Steadman CJ, Phillips SF, Camilleri M, Haddad AC, Hanson RB. Variation of muscle tone in the human colon. *Gastroenterology* 1991;101:373–81.

[211] Rao SS, Kavelock R, Beaty J, Ackerson K, Stumbo P. Effects of fat and carbohydrate meals on colonic motor response. *Gut* 2000;46:205–11.

[212] Sarna SK, Lang IM. Colonic motor response to a meal in dogs. *Am J Physiol* 1989;257: G830–5.

[213] Bassotti G, Betti C, Imbimbo BP, Pelli MA, Morelli A. Colonic motor response to eating: a manometric investigation in proximal and distal portions of the viscus in man. *Am J Gastroenterol* 1989;84:118–22.

[214] Tansy MF, Kendall FM, Murphy JJ. The reflex nature of the gastrocolic propulsive response in the dog. *Surg Gynecol Obstet* 1972;135:404–10.

[215] Tansy MF, Kendall FM, Murphy JJ. A pharmacologic analysis of the gastroileal and gastro-colic reflexes in the dog. *Surg Gynecol Obstet* 1972;135:763–8.

[216] Collman PI, Grundy D, Scratcherd T, Wach RA. Vago-vagal reflexes to the colon of the anaesthetized ferret. *J Physiol* 1984;352:395–402.

[217] Snape WJ, Jr., Wright SH, Battle WM, Cohen S. The gastrocolic response: evidence for a neural mechanism. *Gastroenterology* 1979;77:1235–40.

[218] Bassotti G, Calcara C, Annese V, Fiorella S, Roselli P, Morelli A. Nifedipine and verapamil inhibit the sigmoid colon myoelectric response to eating in healthy volunteers. *Dis Colon Rectum* 1998;41:377–80.

[219] Cremonini F, Camilleri M, McKinzie S, Carlson P, Camilleri CE, Burton D, Thomforde G, Urrutia R, Zinsmeister AR. Effect of CCK-1 antagonist, dexloxiglumide, in female patients with irritable bowel syndrome: a pharmacodynamic and pharmacogenomic study. *Am J Gastroenterol* 2005;100:652–63.

[220] Bassotti G, Imbimbo BP, Betti C, Erbella GS, Pelli MA, Morelli A. Edrophonium chloride for testing colonic contractile activity in man. *Acta Physiol Scand* 1991;141:289–93.

[221] Harris ML, Hobson AR, Hamdy S, Thompson DG, Akkermans LM, Aziz Q. Neurophysiological evaluation of healthy human anorectal sensation. *Am J Physiol Gastrointest Liver Physiol* 2006;291:G950–8.

[222] Thomson A. Anorectal physiology. *Surg Clin North Am* 2002;82:1115–1123.

[223] Rattan S. The internal anal sphincter: regulation of smooth muscle tone and relaxation. *Neurogastroenterol Motil* 2005;17 Suppl 1:50–9.

[224] Dinning PG, Fuentealba SE, Kennedy ML, Lubowski DZ, Cook IJ. Sacral nerve stimulation induces pan-colonic propagating pressure waves and increases defecation frequency in patients with slow-transit constipation. *Colorectal Dis* 2007;9:123–32.

[225] Kamm MA, van der Sijp JR, Lennard-Jones JE. Observations on the characteristics of stimulated defaecation in severe idiopathic constipation. *Int J Colorectal Dis* 1992;7:197–201.

[226] De Schryver AM, Samsom M, Smout AI. Effects of a meal and bisacodyl on colonic motility in healthy volunteers and patients with slow-transit constipation. *Dig Dis Sci* 2003;48:1206–12.

[227] Hardcastle JD, Mann CV. Physical factors in the stimulation of colonic peristalsis. *Gut* 1970;11:41–6.

[228] Kamath PS, Phillips SF, Zinsmeister AR. Short-chain fatty acids stimulate ileal motility in humans. *Gastroenterology* 1988;95:1496–502.

[229] Kamath PS, Hoepfner MT, Phillips SF. Short-chain fatty acids stimulate motility of the canine ileum. *Am J Physiol* 1987;253:G427–33.

[230] Fukumoto S, Tatewaki M, Yamada T, Fujimiya M, Mantyh C, Voss M, Eubanks S, Harris M, Pappas TN, Takahashi T. Short-chain fatty acids stimulate colonic transit via intraluminal 5-HT release in rats. *Am J Physiol Regul Integr Comp Physiol* 2003;284:R1269–76.

[231] Spiller RC, Brown ML, Phillips SF. Decreased fluid tolerance, accelerated transit, and abnormal motility of the human colon induced by oleic acid. *Gastroenterology* 1986;91:100–7.

[232] Dapoigny M, Sarna SK. Effects of physical exercise on colonic motor activity. *Am J Physiol* 1991;260:G646–52.

[233] Holdstock DJ, Misiewicz JJ, Smith T, Rowlands EN. Propulsion (mass movements) in the human colon and its relationship to meals and somatic activity. *Gut* 1970;11:91–9.

[234] Flourie B, Phillips S, Richter H, 3rd, Azpiroz F. Cyclic motility in canine colon: responses to feeding and perfusion. *Dig Dis Sci* 1989;34:1185–92.

[235] Karaus M, Sarna SK, Ammon HV, Wienbeck M. Effects of oral laxatives on colonic motor complexes in dogs. *Gut* 1987;28:1112–9.

[236] Auwerda JJ, Bac DJ, Schouten WR. Circadian rhythm of rectal motor complexes. *Dis Colon Rectum* 2001;44:1328–32.

[237] Ronholt C, Rasmussen OO, Christiansen J. Ambulatory manometric recording of anorectal activity. *Dis Colon Rectum* 1999;42:1551–9.

[238] Kumar D, Williams NS, Waldron D, Wingate DL. Prolonged manometric recording of anorectal motor activity in ambulant human subjects: evidence of periodic activity. *Gut* 1989;30:1007–11.

[239] Orkin BHRKK. The rectal motor complex. *J Gastrointest Motil* 1989;1:5–8.

[240] Orkin BA, Hanson RB, Kelly KA, Phillips SF, Dent J. Human anal motility while fasting, after feeding, and during sleep. *Gastroenterology* 1991;100:1016–23.

[241] Prior A, Fearn UJ, Read NW. Intermittent rectal motor activity: a rectal motor complex? *Gut* 1991;32:1360–3.

[242] Ferrara A, Pemberton JH, Levin KE, Hanson RB. Relationship between anal canal tone and rectal motor activity. *Dis Colon Rectum* 1993;36:337–42.

[243] Taylor BM, Beart RW, Jr., Phillips SF. Longitudinal and radial variations of pressure in the human anal sphincter. *Gastroenterology* 1984;86:693–7.

[244] Rao SS, Welcher K. Periodic rectal motor activity: the intrinsic colonic gatekeeper? *Am J Gastroenterol* 1996;91:890–7.

[245] Lynn PA, Blackshaw LA. In vitro recordings of afferent fibres with receptive fields in the serosa, muscle and mucosa of rat colon. *J Physiol* 1999;518(Pt 1):271–82.

[246] Brierley SM, Jones RC, 3rd, Gebhart GF, Blackshaw LA. Splanchnic and pelvic mechanosensory afferents signal different qualities of colonic stimuli in mice. *Gastroenterology* 2004; 127:166–78.

[247] Lembo T, Munakata J, Naliboff B, Fullerton S, Mayer EA. Sigmoid afferent mechanisms in patients with irritable bowel syndrome. *Dig Dis Sci* 1997;42:1112–20.

[248] Drossman DA, Camilleri M, Mayer EA, Whitehead WE. AGA technical review on irritable bowel syndrome. *Gastroenterology* 2002;123:2108–31.

[249] Mertz HR. Irritable bowel syndrome. *N Engl J Med* 2003;349:2136–46.

[250] Saito YA, Schoenfeld P, Locke GR, 3rd. The epidemiology of irritable bowel syndrome in North America: a systematic review. *Am J Gastroenterol* 2002;97:1910–5.

[251] Chial HJ, Camilleri M. Gender differences in irritable bowel syndrome. *J Gend Specif Med* 2002;5:37–45.

[252] Thompson WG, Longstreth GF, Drossman DA, Heaton KW, Irvine EJ, Muller-Lissner SA. Functional bowel disorders and functional abdominal pain. *Gut* 1999;45(Suppl 2): II43–7.

[253] Longstreth GF, Thompson WG, Chey WD, Houghton LA, Mearin F, Spiller RC. Functional bowel disorders. *Gastroenterology* 2006;130:1480–91.

[254] Camilleri M, McKinzie S, Busciglio I, Low PA, Sweetser S, Burton D, Baxter K, Ryks M, Zinsmeister AR. Prospective study of motor, sensory, psychologic, and autonomic functions in patients with irritable bowel syndrome. *Clin Gastroenterol Hepatol* 2008;6:772–81.

[255] Cann PA, Read NW, Brown C, Hobson N, Holdsworth CD. Irritable bowel syndrome: relationship of disorders in the transit of a single solid meal to symptom patterns. *Gut* 1983; 24:405–11.

[256] Vassallo M, Camilleri M, Phillips SF, Brown ML, Chapman NJ, Thomforde GM. Transit through the proximal colon influences stool weight in the irritable bowel syndrome. *Gastroenterology* 1992;102:102–8.

[257] Horikawa Y, Mieno H, Inoue M, Kajiyama G. Gastrointestinal motility in patients with irritable bowel syndrome studied by using radiopaque markers. *Scand J Gastroenterol* 1999; 34:1190–5.

[258] Bazzocchi G, Ellis J, Villanueva-Meyer J, Reddy SN, Mena I, Snape WJ, Jr. Effect of eating on colonic motility and transit in patients with functional diarrhea. Simultaneous scintigraphic and manometric evaluations. *Gastroenterology* 1991;101:1298–306.

[259] Deiteren A, Camilleri M, Burton D, McKinzie S, Rao A, Zinsmeister AR. Effect of meal ingestion on ileocolonic and colonic transit in health and irritable bowel syndrome. *Dig Dis Sci* 2010;55:384–91.

[260] Manabe N, Wong BS, Camilleri M, Burton D, McKinzie S, Zinsmeister AR. Lower functional gastrointestinal disorders: evidence of abnormal colonic transit in a 287 patient cohort. *Neurogastroenterol Motil* 2010;22:293–e82.

[261] Bouchoucha M, Devroede G, Dorval E, Faye A, Arhan P, Arsac M. Different segmental

transit times in patients with irritable bowel syndrome and "normal" colonic transit time: is there a correlation with symptoms? *Tech Coloproctol* 2006;10:287–96.

[262] Ritchie J. Pain from distension of the pelvic colon by inflating a balloon in the irritable colon syndrome. *Gut* 1973;14:125–32.

[263] Mertz H, Naliboff B, Munakata J, Niazi N, Mayer EA. Altered rectal perception is a biological marker of patients with irritable bowel syndrome. *Gastroenterology* 1995;109:40–52.

[264] Bradette M, Delvaux M, Staumont G, Fioramonti J, Bueno L, Frexinos J. Evaluation of colonic sensory thresholds in IBS patients using a barostat. Definition of optimal conditions and comparison with healthy subjects. *Dig Dis Sci* 1994;39:449–57.

[265] Naliboff BD, Munakata J, Fullerton S, Gracely RH, Kodner A, Harraf F, Mayer EA. Evidence for two distinct perceptual alterations in irritable bowel syndrome. *Gut* 1997;41: 505–12.

[266] Prior A, Read NW. Reduction of rectal sensitivity and post-prandial motility by granisetron, a 5 HT3-receptor antagonist, in patients with irritable bowel syndrome. *Aliment Pharmacol Ther* 1993;7:175–80.

[267] Prior A, Maxton DG, Whorwell PJ. Anorectal manometry in irritable bowel syndrome: differences between diarrhoea and constipation predominant subjects. *Gut* 1990;31: 458–62.

[268] Bassotti G, Chistolini F, Marinozzi G, Morelli A. Abnormal colonic propagated activity in patients with slow transit constipation and constipation-predominant irritable bowel syndrome. *Digestion* 2003;68:178–83.

[269] Bassotti G, de Roberto G, Castellani D, Sediari L, Morelli A. Normal aspects of colorectal motility and abnormalities in slow transit constipation. *World J Gastroenterol* 2005;11: 2691–6.

[270] Hagger R, Kumar D, Benson M, Grundy A. Colonic motor activity in slow-transit idiopathic constipation as identified by 24-h pancolonic ambulatory manometry. *Neurogastroenterol Motil* 2003;15:515–22.

[271] Rao SS, Sadeghi P, Beaty J, Kavlock R. Ambulatory 24-hour colonic manometry in slow-transit constipation. *Am J Gastroenterol* 2004;99:2405–16.

[272] Dinning PG, Bampton PA, Andre J, Kennedy ML, Lubowski DZ, King DW, Cook IJ. Abnormal predefecatory colonic motor patterns define constipation in obstructed defecation. *Gastroenterology* 2004;127:49–56.

[273] Hasler WL, Saad RJ, Rao SS, Wilding GE, Parkman HP, Koch KL, McCallum RW, Kuo B, Sarosiek I, Sitrin MD, Semler JR, Chey WD. Heightened colon motor activity measured by a wireless capsule in patients with constipation: relation to colon transit and IBS. *Am J Physiol Gastrointest Liver Physiol* 2009;297:G1107–14.

[274] Chaudhary NA, Truelove SC. The irritable colon syndrome. A study of the clinical features, predisposing causes, and prognosis in 130 cases. *Q J Med* 1962;31:307–22.

[275] Gwee KA, Graham JC, McKendrick MW, Collins SM, Marshall JS, Walters SJ, Read NW. Psychometric scores and persistence of irritable bowel after infectious diarrhoea. *Lancet* 1996;347:150–3.

[276] Gwee KA, Leong YL, Graham C, McKendrick MW, Collins SM, Walters SJ, Underwood JE, Read NW. The role of psychological and biological factors in postinfective gut dysfunction. *Gut* 1999;44:400–6.

[277] Halvorson HA, Schlett CD, Riddle MS. Postinfectious irritable bowel syndrome—a meta-analysis. *Am J Gastroenterol* 2006;101:1894–9; quiz 1942.

[278] McKendrick MW, Read NW. Irritable bowel syndrome--post salmonella infection. J Infect 1994;29:1–3.

[279] Neal KR, Hebden J, Spiller R. Prevalence of gastrointestinal symptoms six months after bacterial gastroenteritis and risk factors for development of the irritable bowel syndrome: postal survey of patients. *BMJ* 1997;314:779–82.

[280] Parry SD, Stansfield R, Jelley D, Gregory W, Phillips E, Barton JR, Welfare MR. Does bacterial gastroenteritis predispose people to functional gastrointestinal disorders? A prospective, community-based, case-control study. *Am J Gastroenterol* 2003;98:1970–5.

[281] Mearin F, Perez-Oliveras M, Perello A, Vinyet J, Ibanez A, Coderch J, Perona M. Dyspepsia and irritable bowel syndrome after a Salmonella gastroenteritis outbreak: one-year follow-up cohort study. *Gastroenterology* 2005;129:98–104.

[282] Bassotti G, Imbimbo BP, Betti C, Dozzini G, Morelli A. Impaired colonic motor response to eating in patients with slow-transit constipation. *Am J Gastroenterol* 1992;87:504–8.

[283] Bazzocchi G, Ellis J, Villanueva-Meyer J, Jing J, Reddy SN, Mena I, Snape WJ, Jr. Postprandial colonic transit and motor activity in chronic constipation. *Gastroenterology* 1990;98:686–93.

[284] Reynolds JC, Ouyang A, Lee CA, Baker L, Sunshine AG, Cohen S. Chronic severe constipation. Prospective motility studies in 25 consecutive patients. *Gastroenterology* 1987;92:414–20.

[285] O'Brien MD, Camilleri M, von der Ohe MR, Phillips SF, Pemberton JH, Prather CM, Wiste JA, Hanson RB. Motility and tone of the left colon in constipation: a role in clinical practice? *Am J Gastroenterol* 1996;91:2532–8.

[286] Bassotti G, Morelli A, Whitehead WE. Abnormal rectosigmoid myoelectric response to eating in patients with severe idiopathic constipation (slow-transit type). *Dis Colon Rectum* 1992;35:753–6.

[287] Bjornsson ES, Chey WD, Hooper F, Woods ML, Owyang C, Hasler WL. Impaired gastrocolonic response and peristaltic reflex in slow-transit constipation: role of 5-HT(3) pathways. *Am J Physiol Gastrointest Liver Physiol* 2002;283:G400–7.

[288] Daly J, Bergin A, Sun WM, Read NW. Effect of food and anti-cholinergic drugs on the pattern of rectosigmoid contractions. *Gut* 1993;34:799–802.

[289] Mitolo-Chieppa D, Mansi G, Rinaldi R, Montagnani M, Potenza MA, Genualdo M, Serio M, Mitolo CI, Rinaldi M, Altomare DF, Memeo V. Cholinergic stimulation and nonadrenergic, noncholinergic relaxation of human colonic circular muscle in idiopathic chronic constipation. *Dig Dis Sci* 1998;43:2719–26.

[290] Burleigh DE. Evidence for a functional cholinergic deficit in human colonic tissue resected for constipation. *J Pharm Pharmacol* 1988;40:55–7.

[291] Bassotti G, Chiarioni G, Imbimbo BP, Betti C, Bonfante F, Vantini I, Morelli A, Whitehead WE. Impaired colonic motor response to cholinergic stimulation in patients with severe chronic idiopathic (slow transit type) constipation. *Dig Dis Sci* 1993;38:1040–5.

[292] Hoyle CH, Kamm MA, Lennard-Jones JE, Burnstock G. An in vitro electrophysiological study of the colon from patients with idiopathic chronic constipation. *Clin Auton Res* 1992;2:327–33.

[293] Raethjen J, Pilot MA, Knowles C, Warner G, Anand P, Williams N. Selective autonomic and sensory deficits in slow transit constipation. *J Auton Nerv Syst* 1997;66:46–52.

[294] Knowles CH, Scott SM, Wellmer A, Misra VP, Pilot MA, Williams NS, Anand P. Sensory and autonomic neuropathy in patients with idiopathic slow-transit constipation. *Br J Surg* 1999;86:54–60.

[295] Kuiken SD, Lindeboom R, Tytgat GN, Boeckxstaens GE. Relationship between symptoms and hypersensitivity to rectal distension in patients with irritable bowel syndrome. *Aliment Pharmacol Ther* 2005;22:157–64.

[296] Bouin M, Plourde V, Boivin M, Riberdy M, Lupien F, Laganiere M, Verrier P, Poitras P. Rectal distention testing in patients with irritable bowel syndrome: sensitivity, specificity, and predictive values of pain sensory thresholds. *Gastroenterology* 2002;122:1771–7.

[297] Mayer EA, Raybould HE. Role of visceral afferent mechanisms in functional bowel disorders. *Gastroenterology* 1990;99:1688–704.

[298] Mayer EA, Gebhart GF. Basic and clinical aspects of visceral hyperalgesia. *Gastroenterology* 1994;107:271–93.

[299] Mertz H. Role of the brain and sensory pathways in gastrointestinal sensory disorders in humans. *Gut* 2002;51 Suppl 1:i29–33.

[300] Camilleri M, Coulie B, Tack JF. Visceral hypersensitivity: facts, speculations, and challenges. *Gut* 2001;48:125–31.

[301]   Posserud I, Syrous A, Lindstrom L, Tack J, Abrahamsson H, Simren M. Altered rectal perception in irritable bowel syndrome is associated with symptom severity. *Gastroenterology* 2007;133:1113–23.

[302]   Lembo T, Munakata J, Mertz H, Niazi N, Kodner A, Nikas V, Mayer EA. Evidence for the hypersensitivity of lumbar splanchnic afferents in irritable bowel syndrome. *Gastroenterology* 1994;107:1686–96.

[303]   Whitehead WE, Palsson OS. Is rectal pain sensitivity a biological marker for irritable bowel syndrome: psychological influences on pain perception. *Gastroenterology* 1998;115: 1263–71.

[304]   Munakata J, Naliboff B, Harraf F, Kodner A, Lembo T, Chang L, Silverman DH, Mayer EA. Repetitive sigmoid stimulation induces rectal hyperalgesia in patients with irritable bowel syndrome. *Gastroenterology* 1997;112:55–63.

[305]   Chang L, Mayer EA, Labus JS, Schmulson M, Lee OY, Olivas TI, Stains J, Naliboff BD. Effect of sex on perception of rectosigmoid stimuli in irritable bowel syndrome. *Am J Physiol Regul Integr Comp Physiol* 2006;291:R277–84.

[306]   Kanazawa M, Palsson OS, Thiwan SI, Turner MJ, van Tilburg MA, Gangarosa LM, Chitkara DK, Fukudo S, Drossman DA, Whitehead WE. Contributions of pain sensitivity and colonic motility to IBS symptom severity and predominant bowel habits. *Am J Gastroenterol* 2008;103:2550–61.

[307]   Carrasco GA, Van de Kar LD. Neuroendocrine pharmacology of stress. *Eur J Pharmacol* 2003;463:235–72.

[308]   Habib KE, Gold PW, Chrousos GP. Neuroendocrinology of stress. *Endocrinol Metab Clin North Am* 2001;30:695–728; vii–viii.

[309]   Tsigos C, Chrousos GP. Hypothalamic-pituitary-adrenal axis, neuroendocrine factors and stress. *J Psychosom Res* 2002;53:865–71.

[310]   Posserud I, Agerforz P, Ekman R, Bjornsson ES, Abrahamsson H, Simren M. Altered visceral perceptual and neuroendocrine response in patients with irritable bowel syndrome during mental stress. *Gut* 2004;53:1102–8.

[311]   Elsenbruch S, Lovallo WR, Orr WC. Psychological and physiological responses to postprandial mental stress in women with the irritable bowel syndrome. *Psychosom Med* 2001; 63:805–13.

[312]   Dinan TG, Quigley EM, Ahmed SM, Scully P, O'Brien S, O'Mahony L, O'Mahony S, Shanahan F, Keeling PW. Hypothalamic-pituitary-gut axis dysregulation in irritable bowel syndrome: plasma cytokines as a potential biomarker? *Gastroenterology* 2006;130:304–11.

[313]   Elsenbruch S, Orr WC. Diarrhea- and constipation-predominant IBS patients differ in postprandial autonomic and cortisol responses. *Am J Gastroenterol* 2001;96:460–6.

[314] Elsenbruch S, Holtmann G, Oezcan D, Lysson A, Janssen O, Goebel MU, Schedlowski M. Are there alterations of neuroendocrine and cellular immune responses to nutrients in women with irritable bowel syndrome? *Am J Gastroenterol* 2004;99:703–10.

[315] Fukudo S, Nomura T, Hongo M. Impact of corticotropin-releasing hormone on gastro-intestinal motility and adrenocorticotropic hormone in normal controls and patients with irritable bowel syndrome. *Gut* 1998;42:845–9.

[316] Dickhaus B, Mayer EA, Firooz N, Stains J, Conde F, Olivas TI, Fass R, Chang L, Mayer M, Naliboff BD. Irritable bowel syndrome patients show enhanced modulation of visceral perception by auditory stress. *Am J Gastroenterol* 2003;98:135–43.

[317] Bohmelt AH, Nater UM, Franke S, Hellhammer DH, Ehlert U. Basal and stimulated hypothalamic-pituitary-adrenal axis activity in patients with functional gastrointestinal disorders and healthy controls. *Psychosom Med* 2005;67:288–94.

[318] Heitkemper M, Jarrett M, Cain K, Shaver J, Bond E, Woods NF, Walker E. Increased urine catecholamines and cortisol in women with irritable bowel syndrome. *Am J Gastroenterol* 1996;91:906–13.

[319] Heitkemper M, Jarrett M, Cain KC, Burr R, Levy RL, Feld A, Hertig V. Autonomic nervous system function in women with irritable bowel syndrome. *Dig Dis Sci* 2001;46:1276–84.

[320] Cain KC, Jarrett ME, Burr RL, Hertig VL, Heitkemper MM. Heart rate variability is related to pain severity and predominant bowel pattern in women with irritable bowel syndrome. *Neurogastroenterol Motil* 2007;19:110–8.

[321] Chang L, Sundaresh S, Elliott J, Anton PA, Baldi P, Licudine A, Mayer M, Vuong T, Hirano M, Naliboff BD, Ameen VZ, Mayer EA. Dysregulation of the hypothalamic-pituitary-adrenal (HPA) axis in irritable bowel syndrome. *Neurogastroenterol Motil* 2009; 21:149–59.

[322] Tsukamoto K, Nakade Y, Mantyh C, Ludwig K, Pappas TN, Takahashi T. Peripherally administered CRF stimulates colonic motility via central CRF receptors and vagal pathways in conscious rats. *Am J Physiol Regul Integr Comp Physiol* 2006;290:R1537–41.

[323] Tache Y, Monnikes H, Bonaz B, Rivier J. Role of CRF in stress-related alterations of gastric and colonic motor function. *Ann N Y Acad Sci* 1993;697:233–43.

[324] Tache Y, Martinez V, Million M, Wang L. Stress and the gastrointestinal tract III. Stress-related alterations of gut motor function: role of brain corticotropin-releasing factor receptors. *Am J Physiol Gastrointest Liver Physiol* 2001;280:G173–7.

[325] Bach DR, Erdmann G, Schmidtmann M, Monnikes H. Emotional stress reactivity in irritable bowel syndrome. *Eur J Gastroenterol Hepatol* 2006;18:629–36.

[326] Spetalen S, Sandvik L, Blomhoff S, Jacobsen MB. Rectal visceral sensitivity in women with irritable bowel syndrome without psychiatric comorbidity compared with healthy volunteers. *Gastroenterol Res Pract* 2009;2009:130684.

[327] Bennett EJ, Tennant CC, Piesse C, Badcock CA, Kellow JE. Level of chronic life stress predicts clinical outcome in irritable bowel syndrome. *Gut* 1998;43:256–61.

[328] Whitehead WE, Crowell MD, Robinson JC, Heller BR, Schuster MM. Effects of stressful life events on bowel symptoms: subjects with irritable bowel syndrome compared with subjects without bowel dysfunction. *Gut* 1992;33:825–30.

[329] Winston JH, Xu GY, Sarna SK. Adrenergic stimulation mediates visceral hypersensitivity to colorectal distension following heterotypic chronic stress. *Gastroenterology* 2010;138: 294–304 e3.

[330] Bradesi S, Schwetz I, Ennes HS, Lamy CM, Ohning G, Fanselow M, Pothoulakis C, McRoberts JA, Mayer EA. Repeated exposure to water avoidance stress in rats: a new model for sustained visceral hyperalgesia. *Am J Physiol Gastrointest Liver Physiol* 2005;289: G42–53.

[331] Yamaguchi-Shima N, Okada S, Shimizu T, Usui D, Nakamura K, Lu L, Yokotani K. Adrenal adrenaline- and noradrenaline-containing cells and celiac sympathetic ganglia are differentially controlled by centrally administered corticotropin-releasing factor and arginine-vasopressin in rats. *Eur J Pharmacol* 2007;564:94–102.

[332] Morrison SF, Cao WH. Different adrenal sympathetic preganglionic neurons regulate epinephrine and norepinephrine secretion. *Am J Physiol Regul Integr Comp Physiol* 2000;279: R1763–75.

[333] Choudhury BK, Shi XZ, Sarna SK. Norepinephrine mediates the transcriptional effects of heterotypic chronic stress on colonic motor function. *Am J Physiol Gastrointest Liver Physiol* 2009.

[334] Delcroix JD, Valletta JS, Wu C, Hunt SJ, Kowal AS, Mobley WC. NGF signaling in sensory neurons: evidence that early endosomes carry NGF retrograde signals. *Neuron* 2003;39: 69–84.

[335] Leek BF. Abdominal and pelvic visceral receptors. *Br Med Bull* 1977;33:163–8.

[336] Sengupta JN, Gebhart GF. Characterization of mechanosensitive pelvic nerve afferent fibers innervating the colon of the rat. *J Neurophysiol* 1994;71:2046–60.

[337] Hebert MA, Serova LI, Sabban EL. Single and repeated immobilization stress differentially trigger induction and phosphorylation of several transcription factors and mitogen-activated protein kinases in the rat locus coeruleus. *J Neurochem* 2005;95:484–98.

[338] Iwaki K, Sukhatme VP, Shubeita HE, Chien KR. Alpha- and beta-adrenergic stimulation induces distinct patterns of immediate early gene expression in neonatal rat myocardial cells. fos/jun expression is associated with sarcomere assembly; Egr-1 induction is primarily an alpha 1-mediated response. *J Biol Chem* 1990;265:13809–17.

[339] Sabban EL, Kvetnansky R. Stress-triggered activation of gene expression in catecholaminergic systems: dynamics of transcriptional events. *Trends Neurosci* 2001;24:91–8.

[340]   Ueyama T, Yoshida K, Senba E. Emotional stress induces immediate-early gene expression in rat heart via activation of alpha- and beta-adrenoceptors. *Am J Physiol* 1999;277: H1553-61.

[341]   Chitkara DK, van Tilburg MA, Blois-Martin N, Whitehead WE. Early life risk factors that contribute to irritable bowel syndrome in adults: a systematic review. *Am J Gastroenterol* 2008;103:765–74; quiz 775.

[342]   Bengtson MB, Ronning T, Vatn MH, Harris JR. Irritable bowel syndrome in twins: genes and environment. *Gut* 2006;55:1754–9.

[343]   Anand KJ, Runeson B, Jacobson B. Gastric suction at birth associated with long-term risk for functional intestinal disorders in later life. *J Pediatr* 2004;144:449–54.

[344]   Drossman DA, Leserman J, Nachman G, Li ZM, Gluck H, Toomey TC, Mitchell CM. Sexual and physical abuse in women with functional or organic gastrointestinal disorders. *Ann Intern Med* 1990;113:828–33.

[345]   Koloski NA, Talley NJ, Boyce PM. A history of abuse in community subjects with irritable bowel syndrome and functional dyspepsia: the role of other psychosocial variables. *Digestion* 2005;72:86–96.

[346]   Walker EA, Katon WJ, Roy-Byrne PP, Jemelka RP, Russo J. Histories of sexual victimization in patients with irritable bowel syndrome or inflammatory bowel disease. *Am J Psychiatry* 1993;150:1502–6.

[347]   Ross CA. Childhood sexual abuse and psychosomatic symptoms in irritable bowel syndrome. *J Child Sex Abus* 2005;14:27–38.

[348]   Salmon P, Skaife K, Rhodes J. Abuse, dissociation, and somatization in irritable bowel syndrome: towards an explanatory model. *J Behav Med* 2003;26:1–18.

[349]   Talley NJ, Fett SL, Zinsmeister AR, Melton LJ, 3rd. Gastrointestinal tract symptoms and self-reported abuse: a population-based study. *Gastroenterology* 1994;107:1040–9.

[350]   Hislop IG. Childhood deprivation: an antecedent of the irritable bowel syndrome. *Med J Aust* 1979;1:372–4.

[351]   Al-Chaer ED, Kawasaki M, Pasricha PJ. A new model of chronic visceral hypersensitivity in adult rats induced by colon irritation during postnatal development. *Gastroenterology* 2000;119:1276–85.

[352]   Barreau F, Cartier C, Ferrier L, Fioramonti J, Bueno L. Nerve growth factor mediates alterations of colonic sensitivity and mucosal barrier induced by neonatal stress in rats. *Gastroenterology* 2004;127:524–34.

[353]   Coutinho SV, Plotsky PM, Sablad M, Miller JC, Zhou H, Bayati AI, McRoberts JA, Mayer EA. Neonatal maternal separation alters stress-induced responses to viscerosomatic nociceptive stimuli in rat. *Am J Physiol Gastrointest Liver Physiol* 2002;282:G307-16.

[354]   Dunlop SP, Jenkins D, Neal KR, Naesdal J, Borgaonker M, Collins SM, Spiller RC. Randomized, double-blind, placebo-controlled trial of prednisolone in post-infectious irritable bowel syndrome. *Aliment Pharmacol Ther* 2003;18:77–84.

[355]   Choudhury BK, Shi XZ, Sarna SK. Gene plasticity in colonic circular smooth muscle cells underlies motility dysfunction in a model of postinfective IBS. *Am J Physiol Gastrointest Liver Physiol* 2009;296:G632–42.

[356]   Preston DM, Lennard-Jones JE. Severe chronic constipation of young women: 'idiopathic slow transit constipation'. *Gut* 1986;27:41–8.

[357]   Knowles CH, Martin JE. Slow transit constipation: a model of human gut dysmotility. Review of possible aetiologies. *Neurogastroenterol Motil* 2000;12:181–96.

[358]   Xiao ZL, Pricolo V, Biancani P, Behar J. Role of progesterone signaling in the regulation of G-protein levels in female chronic constipation. *Gastroenterology* 2005;128:667–75.

[359]   Cong P, Pricolo V, Biancani P, Behar J. Abnormalities of prostaglandins and cyclooxygenase enzymes in female patients with slow-transit constipation. *Gastroenterology* 2007;133: 445–53.

[360]   Cheng L, Pricolo V, Biancani P, Behar J. Overexpression of progesterone receptor B increases sensitivity of human colon muscle cells to progesterone. *Am J Physiol Gastrointest Liver Physiol* 2008;295:G493–502.

[361]   Lyford GL, He CL, Soffer E, Hull TL, Strong SA, Senagore AJ, Burgart LJ, Young-Fadok T, Szurszewski JH, Farrugia G. Pan-colonic decrease in interstitial cells of Cajal in patients with slow transit constipation. *Gut* 2002;51:496–501.

[362]   Tong WD, Liu BH, Zhang LY, Zhang SB, Lei Y. Decreased interstitial cells of Cajal in the sigmoid colon of patients with slow transit constipation. *Int J Colorectal Dis* 2004;19: 467–73.

[363]   Wedel T, Spiegler J, Soellner S, Roblick UJ, Schiedeck TH, Bruch HP, Krammer HJ. Enteric nerves and interstitial cells of Cajal are altered in patients with slow-transit constipation and megacolon. *Gastroenterology* 2002;123:1459–67.

[364]   Yu CS, Kim HC, Hong HK, Chung DH, Kim HJ, Kang GH, Kim JC. Evaluation of myenteric ganglion cells and interstitial cells of Cajal in patients with chronic idiopathic constipation. *Int J Colorectal Dis* 2002;17:253–8.

[365]   Zhang Y, Carmichael SA, Wang XY, Huizinga JD, Paterson WG. Neurotransmission in lower esophageal sphincter of W/Wv mutant mice. *Am J Physiol Gastrointest Liver Physiol* 2010;298:G14–24.

[366]   Sarna S, Latimer P, Campbell D, Waterfall WE. Effect of stress, meal and neostigmine on rectosigmoid electrical control activity (ECA) in normals and in irritable bowel syndrome patients. *Dig Dis Sci* 1982;27:582–91.

[367] Goldin E, Karmeli F, Selinger Z, Rachmilewitz D. Colonic substance P levels are increased in ulcerative colitis and decreased in chronic severe constipation. *Dig Dis Sci* 1989;34: 754–7.

[368] Lincoln J, Crowe R, Kamm MA, Burnstock G, Lennard-Jones JE. Serotonin and 5-hydroxyindoleacetic acid are increased in the sigmoid colon in severe idiopathic constipation. *Gastroenterology* 1990;98:1219–25.

[369] Tzavella K, Riepl RL, Klauser AG, Voderholzer WA, Schindlbeck NE, Muller-Lissner SA. Decreased substance P levels in rectal biopsies from patients with slow transit constipation. *Eur J Gastroenterol Hepatol* 1996;8:1207–11.

[370] Park HJ, Kamm MA, Abbasi AM, Talbot IC. Immunohistochemical study of the colonic muscle and innervation in idiopathic chronic constipation. *Dis Colon Rectum* 1995;38: 509–13.

[371] Koch TR, Carney JA, Go L, Go VL. Idiopathic chronic constipation is associated with decreased colonic vasoactive intestinal peptide. *Gastroenterology* 1988;94:300–10.

[372] Dolk A, Broden G, Holmstrom B, Johansson C, Schultzberg M. Slow transit chronic constipation (Arbuthnot Lane's disease). An immunohistochemical study of neuropeptide-containing nerves in resected specimens from the large bowel. *Int J Colorectal Dis* 1990; 5:181–7.

[373] Sjolund K, Fasth S, Ekman R, Hulten L, Jiborn H, Nordgren S, Sundler F. Neuropeptides in idiopathic chronic constipation (slow transit constipation). *Neurogastroenterol Motil* 1997;9:143–50.

[374] Cortesini C, Cianchi F, Infantino A, Lise M. Nitric oxide synthase and VIP distribution in enteric nervous system in idiopathic chronic constipation. *Dig Dis Sci* 1995;40:2450–5.

[375] O'Sullivan BP, Freedman SD. Cystic fibrosis. *Lancet* 2009;373:1891–904.

[376] Vencesla A, Fuentes-Prior P, Baena M, Quintana M, Baiget M, Tizzano EF. Severe haemophilia A in a female resulting from an inherited gross deletion and a de novo codon deletion in the F8 gene. *Haemophilia* 2008;14:1094–8.

[377] Steinberg MH. Sickle cell anemia, the first molecular disease: overview of molecular etiology, pathophysiology, and therapeutic approaches. *Sci World J* 2008;8:1295–324.

[378] King Meae. *The Genetic Bases of Common Diseases*, Oxford University Press. 1992.

[379] Childs B. A logic of disease. In: *The Metabolic and Molecular Bases of Inherited Disease*, 7th edition, Scriver, CR et al. eds. McGraw-Hill. 1995:229–257.

[380] Howard R, Rabins PV, Seeman MV, Jeste DV. Late-onset schizophrenia and very-late-onset schizophrenia-like psychosis: an international consensus. The International Late-Onset Schizophrenia Group. *Am J Psychiatry* 2000;157:172–8.

[381] Davis CD, Uthus EO. DNA methylation, cancer susceptibility, and nutrient interactions. *Exp Biol Med* (Maywood) 2004;229:988–95.

[382] Adcock IM, Tsaprouni L, Bhavsar P, Ito K. Epigenetic regulation of airway inflammation. *Curr Opin Immunol* 2007;19:694–700.

[383] Wilson AG. Epigenetic regulation of gene expression in the inflammatory response and relevance to common diseases. *J Periodontol* 2008;79:1514–9.

[384] Barnes PJ, Adcock IM, Ito K. Histone acetylation and deacetylation: importance in inflammatory lung diseases. *Eur Respir J* 2005;25:552–63.

[385] Hitchler MJ, Domann FE. Metabolic defects provide a spark for the epigenetic switch in cancer. *Free Radic Biol Med* 2009;47:115–27.

[386] Valinluck V, Sowers LC. Inflammation-mediated cytosine damage: a mechanistic link between inflammation and the epigenetic alterations in human cancers. *Cancer Res* 2007; 67:5583–6.

[387] Petronis A. Human morbid genetics revisited: relevance of epigenetics. Trends Genet 2001; 17:142–6.

[388] Barker DJ, Osmond C. Infant mortality, childhood nutrition, and ischaemic heart disease in England and Wales. *Lancet* 1986;1:1077–81.

[389] Allfrey VG, Faulkner R, Mirsky AE. Acetylation and Methylation of Histones and Their Possible Role in the Regulation of Rna Synthesis. *Proc Natl Acad Sci U S A* 1964;51: 786–94.

[390] Pogo BG, Allfrey VG, Mirsky AE. RNA synthesis and histone acetylation during the course of gene activation in lymphocytes. *Proc Natl Acad Sci U S A* 1966;55:805–12.

[391] Wu J, Grunstein M. 25 years after the nucleosome model: chromatin modifications. *Trends Biochem Sci* 2000;25:619–23.

[392] Luger K, Mader AW, Richmond RK, Sargent DF, Richmond TJ. Crystal structure of the nucleosome core particle at 2.8 A resolution. *Nature* 1997;389:251–60.

[393] Bhaumik SR, Smith E, Shilatifard A. Covalent modifications of histones during development and disease pathogenesis. *Nat Struct Mol Biol* 2007;14:1008–16.

[394] Haberland M, Montgomery RL, Olson EN. The many roles of histone deacetylases in development and physiology: implications for disease and therapy. *Nat Rev Genet* 2009; 10:32–42.

[395] Bandyopadhyay K, Baneres JL, Martin A, Blonski C, Parello J, Gjerset RA. Spermidinyl-CoA-based HAT inhibitors block DNA repair and provide cancer-specific chemo- and radiosensitization. *Cell Cycle* 2009;8.

[396] Bandyopadhyay K, Baneres JL, Martin A, Blonski C, Parello J, Gjerset RA. Spermidinyl-CoA-based HAT inhibitors block DNA repair and provide cancer-specific chemo- and radiosensitization. *Cell Cycle* 2009;8:2779–88.

[397] Guil S, Esteller M. DNA methylomes, histone codes and miRNAs: tying it all together. *Int J Biochem Cell Biol* 2009;41:87–95.

[398]   Hodl M, Basler K. Transcription in the absence of histone H3.3. *Curr Biol* 2009;19: 1221–6.

[399]   Bird A. DNA methylation patterns and epigenetic memory. *Genes Dev* 2002;16:6–21.

[400]   Zilberman D, Gehring M, Tran RK, Ballinger T, Henikoff S. Genome-wide analysis of Arabidopsis thaliana DNA methylation uncovers an interdependence between methylation and transcription. *Nat Genet* 2007;39:61–9.

[401]   Deng G, Chen A, Pong E, Kim YS. Methylation in hMLH1 promoter interferes with its binding to transcription factor CBF and inhibits gene expression. *Oncogene* 2001;20: 7120–7.

[402]   Siedlecki P, Zielenkiewicz P. Mammalian DNA methyltransferases. Acta Biochim Pol 2006;53:245–56.

[403]   Dong A, Yoder JA, Zhang X, Zhou L, Bestor TH, Cheng X. Structure of human DNMT2, an enigmatic DNA methyltransferase homolog that displays denaturant-resistant binding to DNA. *Nucleic Acids Res* 2001;29:439–48.

[404]   Kay L. Prevalence, incidence and prognosis of gastrointestinal symptoms in a random sample of an elderly population. *Age Ageing* 1994;23:146–9.

[405]   Agreus L, Svardsudd K, Nyren O, Tibblin G. Irritable bowel syndrome and dyspepsia in the general population: overlap and lack of stability over time. *Gastroenterology* 1995;109: 671–80.

[406]   Read NW. Diarrhee motrice. *Clin Gastroenterol* 1986;15:657–86.

[407]   Rao SS, Holdsworth CD, Read NW. Symptoms and stool patterns in patients with ulcerative colitis. *Gut* 1988;29:342–5.

[408]   Rao SS, Read NW, Brown C, Bruce C, Holdsworth CD. Studies on the mechanism of bowel disturbance in ulcerative colitis. *Gastroenterology* 1987;93:934–40.

[409]   Kern F, Jr., Almy TP, Abbot FK, Bogdonoff MD. The motility of the distal colon in nonspecific ulcerative colitis. *Gastroenterology* 1951;19:492–503.

[410]   Spriggs EA, Code CF, Bargen JA, Curtiss RK, Hightower NC, Jr. Motility of the pelvic colon and rectum of normal persons and patients with ulcerative colitis. *Gastroenterology* 1951;19:480–91.

[411]   Jalan KN, Walker RJ, Prescott RJ, Butterworth ST, Smith AN, Sircus W. Faecal stasis and diverticular disease in ulcerative colitis. *Gut* 1970;11:688–96.

[412]   Lennard-Jones JE, Langman MJ, Jones FA. Faecal stasis in proctocolitis. *Gut* 1962;3: 301–5.

[413]   Annese V, Bassotti G, Napolitano G, Usai P, Andriulli A, Vantrappen G. Gastrointestinal motility disorders in patients with inactive Crohn's disease. *Scand J Gastroenterol* 1997; 32:1107–17.

[414] Loening-Baucke V, Metcalf AM, Shirazi S. Anorectal manometry in active and quiescent ulcerative colitis. *Am J Gastroenterol* 1989;84:892–7.

[415] Snape WJ, Jr. The role of a colonic motility disturbance in ulcerative colitis. *Keio J Med* 1991;40:6–8.

[416] Connell AM. The motility of the pelvic colon. II. Paradoxical motility in diarrhoea and constipation. *Gut* 1962;3:342–8.

[417] Collins SM. The immunomodulation of enteric neuromuscular function: implications for motility and inflammatory disorders. *Gastroenterology* 1996;111:1683–99.

[418] Lium R, Porter JE. Observations on the etiology of ulcerative colitis: III. The distribution of lesions and its possible significance. *Am J Pathol* 1939;15:73–78 3.

[419] Jouet P, Sarna SK, Singaram C, Ryan RP, Hillard CJ, Telford GL, Fink J, Henderson JD. Immunocytes and abnormal gastrointestinal motor activity during ileitis in dogs. *Am J Physiol* 1995;269:G913–24.

[420] Otterson MF, Sarna SK, Leming SC, Moulder JE, Fink JG. Effects of fractionated doses of ionizing radiation on colonic motor activity. *Am J Physiol* 1992;263:G518–26.

[421] Belaiche J, Louis E, D'Haens G, Cabooter M, Naegels S, De Vos M, Fontaine F, Schurmans P, Baert F, De Reuck M, Fiasse R, Holvoet J, Schmit A, Van Outryve M. Acute lower gastrointestinal bleeding in Crohn's disease: characteristics of a unique series of 34 patients. Belgian IBD Research Group. *Am J Gastroenterol* 1999;94:2177–81.

[422] Kostka R, Lukas M. Massive, life-threatening bleeding in Crohn's disease. *Acta Chir Belg* 2005;105:168–74.

[423] Farthing MJ, Lennard-jones JE. Sensibility of the rectum to distension and the anorectal distension reflex in ulcerative colitis. *Gut* 1978;19:64–9.

[424] Chang L, Munakata J, Mayer EA, Schmulson MJ, Johnson TD, Bernstein CN, Saba L, Naliboff B, Anton PA, Matin K. Perceptual responses in patients with inflammatory and functional bowel disease. *Gut* 2000;47:497–505.

[425] Bernstein CN, Niazi N, Robert M, Mertz H, Kodner A, Munakata J, Naliboff B, Mayer EA. Rectal afferent function in patients with inflammatory and functional intestinal disorders. *Pain* 1996;66:151–61.

[426] Delafoy L, Raymond F, Doherty AM, Eschalier A, Diop L. Role of nerve growth factor in the trinitrobenzene sulfonic acid-induced colonic hypersensitivity. *Pain* 2003;105:489–97.

[427] Woolf CJ, Safieh-Garabedian B, Ma QP, Crilly P, Winter J. Nerve growth factor contributes to the generation of inflammatory sensory hypersensitivity. *Neuroscience* 1994;62:327–31.

[428] Sengupta JN, Snider A, Su X, Gebhart GF. Effects of kappa opioids in the inflamed rat colon. *Pain* 1999;79:175–85.

[429] Hughes PA, Brierley SM, Martin CM, Brookes SJ, Linden DR, Blackshaw LA. Post-inflammatory colonic afferent sensitisation: different subtypes, different pathways and different time courses. *Gut* 2009;58:1333–41.

[430] Agostini S, Eutamene H, Broccardo M, Improta G, Petrella C, Theodorou V, Bueno L. Peripheral anti-nociceptive effect of nociceptin/orphanin FQ in inflammation and stress-induced colonic hyperalgesia in rats. *Pain* 2009;141:292–9.

[431] Zhou Q, Price DD, Caudle RM, Verne GN. Visceral and somatic hypersensitivity in TNBS-induced colitis in rats. *Dig Dis Sci* 2008;53:429–35.

[432] Ohashi K, Sato Y, Iwata H, Kawai M, Kurebayashi Y. Colonic mast cell infiltration in rats with TNBS-induced visceral hypersensitivity. *J Vet Med Sci* 2007;69:1223–8.

[433] Elson CO, Sartor RB, Tennyson GS, Riddell RH. Experimental models of inflammatory bowel disease. *Gastroenterology* 1995;109:1344–67.

[434] Snape WJ, Jr., Williams R, Hyman PE. Defect in colonic smooth muscle contraction in patients with ulcerative colitis. *Am J Physiol* 1991;261:G987–91.

[435] Vrees MD, Pricolo VE, Potenti FM, Cao W. Abnormal motility in patients with ulcerative colitis: the role of inflammatory cytokines. *Arch Surg* 2002;137:439–45; discussion 445–6.

[436] Vermillion DL, Huizinga JD, Riddell RH, Collins SM. Altered small intestinal smooth muscle function in Crohn's disease. *Gastroenterology* 1993;104:1692–9.

[437] Hosseini JM, Goldhill JM, Bossone C, Pineiro-Carrero V, Shea-Donohue T. Progressive alterations in circular smooth muscle contractility in TNBS-induced colitis in rats. *Neurogastroenterol Motil* 1999;11:347–56.

[438] Kinoshita K, Sato K, Hori M, Ozaki H, Karaki H. Decrease in activity of smooth muscle L-type Ca2+ channels and its reversal by NF-kappaB inhibitors in Crohn's colitis model. *Am J Physiol Gastrointest Liver Physiol* 2003;285:G483–93.

[439] Kiyosue M, Fujisawa M, Kinoshita K, Hori M, Ozaki H. Different susceptibilities of spontaneous rhythmicity and myogenic contractility to intestinal muscularis inflammation in the hapten-induced colitis. *Neurogastroenterol Motil* 2006;18:1019–30.

[440] Koch TR, Carney JA, Go VL, Szurszewski JH. Spontaneous contractions and some electrophysiologic properties of circular muscle from normal sigmoid colon and ulcerative colitis. *Gastroenterology* 1988;95:77–84.

[441] Shi XZ, Pazdrak K, Saada N, Dai B, Palade P, Sarna SK. Negative transcriptional regulation of human colonic smooth muscle Cav1.2 channels by p50 and p65 subunits of nuclear factor-kappaB. *Gastroenterology* 2005;129:1518–32.

[442] Pazdrak K, Shi XZ, Sarna SK. TNFalpha suppresses human colonic circular smooth muscle cell contractility by SP1- and NF-kappaB-mediated induction of ICAM-1. *Gastroenterology* 2004;127:1096–109.

[443] Shi XZ, Lindholm PF, Sarna SK. NF-kappa B activation by oxidative stress and inflammation suppresses contractility in colonic circular smooth muscle cells. *Gastroenterology* 2003; 124:1369–80.

[444] Lee EY, Stenson WF, DeSchryver-Kecskemeti K. Thickening of muscularis mucosae in Crohn's disease. *Mod Pathol* 1991;4:87–90.

[445] Gaudio E, Taddei G, Vetuschi A, Sferra R, Frieri G, Ricciardi G, Caprilli R. Dextran sulfate sodium (DSS) colitis in rats: clinical, structural, and ultrastructural aspects. *Dig Dis Sci* 1999;44:1458–75.

[446] Shi XZ, Winston JH, Sarna SK. Differential Immune and Genetic Responses in Rat Models of Crohn's Colitis and Ulcerative Colitis. *Am J Physiol Gastrointest Liver Physiol* 2010.

[447] Pravda J. Radical induction theory of ulcerative colitis. *World J Gastroenterol* 2005;11: 2371–84.

[448] Garcia-Lafuente A, Antolin M, Guarner F, Crespo E, Salas A, Forcada P, Laguarda M, Gavalda J, Baena JA, Vilaseca J, Malagelada JR. Incrimination of anaerobic bacteria in the induction of experimental colitis. *Am J Physiol* 1997;272:G10–5.

[449] Fukata M, Michelsen KS, Eri R, Thomas LS, Hu B, Lukasek K, Nast CC, Lechago J, Xu R, Naiki Y, Soliman A, Arditi M, Abreu MT. Toll-like receptor-4 is required for intestinal response to epithelial injury and limiting bacterial translocation in a murine model of acute colitis. *Am J Physiol Gastrointest Liver Physiol* 2005;288:G1055–65.

[450] Rakoff-Nahoum S, Paglino J, Eslami-Varzaneh F, Edberg S, Medzhitov R. Recognition of commensal microflora by toll-like receptors is required for intestinal homeostasis. *Cell* 2004;118:229–41.

[451] Araki Y, Sugihara H, Hattori T. In vitro effects of dextran sulfate sodium on a Caco-2 cell line and plausible mechanisms for dextran sulfate sodium-induced colitis. *Oncol Rep* 2006;16:1357–62.

[452] Vetuschi A, Latella G, Sferra R, Caprilli R, Gaudio E. Increased proliferation and apoptosis of colonic epithelial cells in dextran sulfate sodium-induced colitis in rats. *Dig Dis Sci* 2002;47:1447–57.

[453] Kitajima S, Takuma S, Morimoto M. Changes in colonic mucosal permeability in mouse colitis induced with dextran sulfate sodium. *Exp Anim* 1999;48:137–43.

[454] Kitajima S, Morimoto M, Sagara E, Shimizu C, Ikeda Y. Dextran sodium sulfate-induced colitis in germ-free IQI/Jic mice. *Exp Anim* 2001;50:387–95.

[455] Dieleman LA, Ridwan BU, Tennyson GS, Beagley KW, Bucy RP, Elson CO. Dextran sulfate sodium-induced colitis occurs in severe combined immunodeficient mice. *Gastroenterology* 1994;107:1643–52.

[456] Anitha M, Joseph I, Ding X, Torre ER, Sawchuk MA, Mwangi S, Hochman S, Sitaraman

SV, Anania F, Srinivasan S. Characterization of fetal and postnatal enteric neuronal cell lines with improvement in intestinal neural function. *Gastroenterology* 2008;134:1424–35.

[457]   Villanacci V, Bassotti G, Nascimbeni R, Antonelli E, Cadei M, Fisogni S, Salerni B, Geboes K. Enteric nervous system abnormalities in inflammatory bowel diseases. *Neurogastroenterol Motil* 2008;20:1009–16.

[458]   Belai A, Boulos PB, Robson T, Burnstock G. Neurochemical coding in the small intestine of patients with Crohn's disease. *Gut* 1997;40:767–74.

[459]   Ohlsson B, Veress B, Lindgren S, Sundkvist G. Enteric ganglioneuritis and abnormal interstitial cells of Cajal: features of inflammatory bowel disease. *Inflamm Bowel Dis* 2007;13: 721–6.

[460]   Cook MG, Dixon MF. An analysis of the reliability of detection and diagnostic value of various pathological features in Crohn's disease and ulcerative colitis. *Gut* 1973;14:255–62.

[461]   Siemers PT, Dobbins WO, 3rd. The Meissner plexus in Crohn's disease of the colon. *Surg Gynecol Obstet* 1974;138:39–42.

[462]   Sanovic S, Lamb DP, Blennerhassett MG. Damage to the enteric nervous system in experimental colitis. *Am J Pathol* 1999;155:1051–7.

[463]   Collins SM, Blennerhassett PA, Blennerhassett MG, Vermillion DL. Impaired acetylcholine release from the myenteric plexus of Trichinella-infected rats. *Am J Physiol* 1989;257: G898–903.

[464]   Davis KA, Masella J, Blennerhassett MG. Acetylcholine metabolism in the inflamed rat intestine. *Exp Neurol* 1998;152:251–8.

[465]   Swain MG, Blennerhassett PA, Collins SM. Impaired sympathetic nerve function in the inflamed rat intestine. *Gastroenterology* 1991;100:675–82.

[466]   Lomax AE, Mawe GM, Sharkey KA. Synaptic facilitation and enhanced neuronal excitability in the submucosal plexus during experimental colitis. *J Physiol* 2005.

[467]   Linden DR, Sharkey KA, Mawe GM. Enhanced excitability of myenteric AH neurones in the inflamed guinea-pig distal colon. *J Physiol* 2003;547:589–601.

[468]   Goyal RK, Chaudhury A. Mounting evidence against the role of ICC in neurotransmission to smooth muscle in the gut. *Am J Physiol Gastrointest Liver Physiol* 2010;298:G10–3.

[469]   Painter NBD. Diverticular disease of the colon, a 20th century problem. *Clin Gastroenterol* 1975;4:2–21.

[470]   Whiteway J, Morson, BC. Pathology of the aging - diverticular disease. *Clin Gastroenterol* 1985;14:829–846.

[471]   Connell AM. Pathogenesis of diverticular disease of the colon. *Adv Intern Med* 1977;22: 377–95.

[472] Almy TP, Howell DA. Medical progress. Diverticular disease of the colon. *N Engl J Med* 1980;302:324–31.

[473] Simpson J, Sundler F, Humes DJ, Jenkins D, Scholefield JH, Spiller RC. Post inflammatory damage to the enteric nervous system in diverticular disease and its relationship to symptoms. *Neurogastroenterol Motil* 2009;21:847–e58.

[474] Simpson J, Neal KR, Scholefield JH, Spiller RC. Patterns of pain in diverticular disease and the influence of acute diverticulitis. *Eur J Gastroenterol Hepatol* 2003;15:1005–10.

[475] Parks TG. Natural history of diverticular disease of the colon. *Clin Gastroenterol* 1975;4: 53–69.

[476] Cortesini C, Pantalone D. Usefulness of colonic motility study in identifying patients at risk for complicated diverticular disease. *Dis Colon Rectum* 1991;34:339–42.

[477] Morson BC. The muscle abnormality in diverticular disease of the colon. *Proc R Soc Med* 1963;56:798–800.

[478] Hughes LE. Postmortem survey of diverticular disease of the colon. II. The muscular abnormality of the sigmoid colon. *Gut* 1969;10:344–51.

[479] Bassotti G, Battaglia E, De Roberto G, Morelli A, Tonini M, Villanacci V. Alterations in colonic motility and relationship to pain in colonic diverticulosis. *Clin Gastroenterol Hepatol* 2005;3:248–53.

[480] Trotman IF, Misiewicz JJ. Sigmoid motility in diverticular disease and the irritable bowel syndrome. *Gut* 1988;29:218–22.

[481] Painter NS, Truelove SC. The Intraluminal Pressure Patterns in Diverticulosis of the Colon.3. The effect of prostigmine. Iv. The effect of pethidine and probanthine. *Gut* 1964; 5:365–73.

[482] Arfwidsson S, Knock NG, Lehmann L, Winberg T. Pathogenesis of multiple diverticula of the sogmoid colon in diverticular disease. *Acta Chir Scand Suppl* 1964;63(Suppl 342) 1–68.

[483] Brodribb AJ, Humphreys DM. Diverticular disease: three studies. Part I—Relation to other disorders and fibre intake. *Br Med J* 1976;1:424–5.

[484] Gear JS, Ware A, Fursdon P, Mann JI, Nolan DJ, Brodribb AJ, Vessey MP. Symptomless diverticular disease and intake of dietary fibre. *Lancet* 1979;1:511–4.

[485] Burkitt DP, Walker AR, Painter NS. Effect of dietary fibre on stools and the transit-times, and its role in the causation of disease. *Lancet* 1972;2:1408–12.

[486] Watters DA, Smith AN, Eastwood MA, Anderson KC, Elton RA, Mugerwa JW. Mechanical properties of the colon: comparison of the features of the African and European colon in vitro. *Gut* 1985;26:384–92.

[487]   Slack WW. The anatomy, pathology, and some clinical features of divericulitis of the colon. *Br J Surg* 1962;50:185–90.

[488]   Simpson J, Scholefield JH, Spiller RC. Pathogenesis of colonic diverticula. *Br J Surg* 2002; 89:546–54.

[489]   Smith AN, Shepherd J, Eastwood MA. Pressure changes after balloon distension of the colon wall in diverticular disease. *Gut* 1981;22:841–4.

[490]   Parks TG. Rectal and colonic studies after resection of the sigmoid for diverticular disease. *Gut* 1970;11:121–5.

[491]   Beighton PH, Murdoch JL, Votteler T. Gastrointestinal complications of the Ehlers-Danlos syndrome. *Gut* 1969;10:1004–8.

[492]   Eliashar R, Sichel JY, Biron A, Dano I. Multiple gastrointestinal complications in Marfan syndrome. *Postgrad Med J* 1998;74:495–7.

[493]   Clemens CH, Samsom M, Roelofs J, van Berge Henegouwen GP, Smout AJ. Colorectal visceral perception in diverticular disease. *Gut* 2004;53:717–22.

[494]   Humes DJ, Simpson J, Neal KR, Scholefield JH, Spiller RC. Psychological and colonic factors in painful diverticulosis. *Br J Surg* 2008;95:195–8.

[495]   Sarna SK. In vivo myoelectric activity: methods, analysis, and interpretation. *Am Physiol Soc* 1989.

[496]   Sarna SK. *Myoelectrical and Contractile Activities of the Gastrointestinal Tract.* B.C., Decker, Inc, 2002.

[497]   Lembo A, Camilleri M. Chronic constipation. *N Engl J Med* 2003;349:1360–8.

[498]   Waldron DJ, Kumar D, Hallan RI, Wingate DL, Williams NS. Evidence for motor neuropathy and reduced filling of the rectum in chronic intractable constipation. *Gut* 1990;31: 1284–8.